ANNA RICHARDSON
MINDOVER
FATTER

SEE Yourself Slim
THINK Yourself Slim
EAT Yourself Slim

headline

First published in 2015 by HEADLINE PUBLISHING GROUP

1

Cataloguing in Publication Data is available from the British Library

ISBN 978 1 4722 2624 2

Recipes created by Louisa Carter and Charlotte Simpkins
Hypnotherapy consultant: Marisa Peer
Psychology consultant: Dr Christy Fergusson
Project edited by Emma Tait
Design and art direction by Smith and Gilmour
Photography by Matt Russell
Food styling by Emma Marsden
Hair and make-up by Clare Turner
Props styling by Linder Berlin

Printed and bound in Germany by Mohn Media

Headline's policy is to use papers that are natural, renewable and recyclable products and made from wood grown in well-managed forests and other controlled sources. The logging and manufacturing processes are expected to conform to the environmental regulations of the country of origin.

HEADLINE PUBLISHING GROUP
An Hachette UK Company
338 Euston Road, London NW1 3BH

www.mindoverfatterdownload.co.uk

Neither this diet nor any other diet program should be followed without first consulting a health care professional. If you have any special conditions requiring attention, you should consult with your health care professional regularly regarding possible modification of the program contained in this book.

CONTENTS

Introduction: Eating My Words 6
How This Book Works: The Three-Step Programme 16
It's Not Your Fault You're Fat 20
Diets Over the Decades 24
So What's Eating You? 28
The *Mind Over Fatter* Timeline Regression Download 40
Getting Ready to Change... Yourself 42
Do you See it, Hear it, Feel it or Think it? 50

★ ★ ★

STEP 1: SEE YOURSELF SLIM 55
The Power of the Subconscious Mind 56
The Power of Hypnosis 66
The *Mind Over Fatter* Hypnotherapy Download 68

★ ★ ★

STEP 2: THINK YOURSELF SLIM 71
The Seven Secrets of Slim 72

★ ★ ★

STEP 3: EAT YOURSELF SLIM 89
Feeding Your Body 90
Food on the Brain 92
A Mindful Kitchen 96
The Mind Over Fatter 14-day Healthy-eating Plan 100
Breakfasts 105
Lunches 125
Dinners 159
Soups 195
Snacks 205

Index 218
References 223
A Big Thank You 224

EATING MY WORDS

You'd think by now I'd know a thing or two about food and dieting. After all, I've presented seven series on TV about diets; written my own bestselling diet book *Body Blitz Diet;* and lost over two stone after following my own diet. Yup, like a London cabby doing The Knowledge, I'm a walking A–Z when it comes to weight loss. From Atkins to alkaline, fasting to foraging, and detox to Dukan – I've done the lot. A quick count of the books on my kitchen shelf shows that I've collected over 20 titles on weight loss. But they're nestled between hardback recipe books full of high-calorie cakes. They're all bibles to my belly in their different ways, and show the schizophrenic nature of weight control. I'm a diet guru alright, but I'm also still a normal girl in love with her food – and it's always, always been a battle.

The fact is, many of us struggle every day to overcome our overeating. Despite our best intentions, we fall off the diet wagon again and again, and end up losing control of ourselves as well as the scales. It's a sad fact that women spend up to 17 years of their lives on a diet… and yet 99 per cent of us fail within the first year of trying.

Buy *why*? Is it a lack of willpower? Or just a big fat plate of denial that's causing this diet derailment? And, more importantly, does this sound anything like you?

Well, I think I know the answer. And the chances are that if you've got this book in your hands then you want to know the answer too. So I'm going to ask you to come on a journey with me. It's a trip through my past, present and future. And listen carefully, because once we're done, we're both going to do it again. But this time, it'll be your journey. And believe me, it's going to be an adventure.

So strap yourself in because this book might just change your life… in more ways than you think.

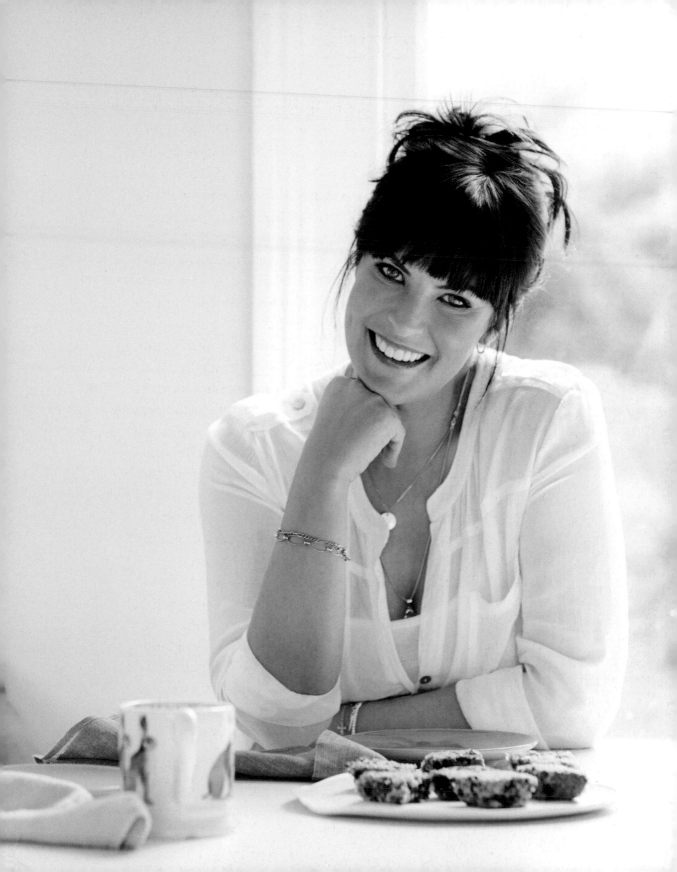

LOOK BACK IN HUNGER

How often have you heard someone say 'Leave the past behind you', 'There's no point looking back' or 'What's done is done'? I'm a big fan of not dwelling too deeply in the murky waters of what's gone before. After all, it's full of regrets isn't it? And yet… and yet… the past is also a great teacher. And you'd be amazed at what we've forgotten to learn. Wasn't it the great philosopher Kierkegaard who said life can only be understood backwards? I know, I get it, this is getting a bit heavy for a book on portion control, but let me explain what I mean.

A few years ago, I was presenting a TV series called *Supersize v Superskinny* and my job as an immersive journalist was to investigate extreme diets and then try them out for size – in order to reduce my size, if you see what I mean. Frankly, I thought it was a bit of a cheek. Because, in my head at least, I was a svelte size 10 supermodel with the looks of a panther and the body of an Olympian. The reality? Well, the reality was a different story.

I hadn't actually weighed myself for over seven years. So when I was asked to strip down to my pants and hop on the scales *on camera* time quite literally stood still. In slow motion I looked down at my toes, clocked the dial beneath me and sucked in a long, horrible gasp. A silent scream surged up from my overhanging belly. The scales read 11 stone and 7 pounds (73 kilograms). I was pretty sure Kate Moss didn't weigh 11 stone and 7 pounds. I'd put money on Angelina Jolie not weighing 11 stone and 7 pounds. Were the scales wrong? Should I put them on a hard surface and try again? And then the truth hit me as I stood in my support knickers, my size 16 (with the label cut out) leggings crumpled on the floor beside me. Could it be that I was actually… *overweight*?!

One week later, I met an amazing woman called Marisa Peer. Marisa is a well-known hypnotherapist and a specialist in weight loss. As part of the show, I was asked to undergo one session of hypnotherapy with her and report back on whether it was effective for losing weight. I'll be honest with you. The crew and I stood outside the house, sceptical TV journalists, convinced that hypnotherapy was a load of old hokum and I'd end up believing I was Cleopatra in a past life. 'Still,' I thought, 'I suppose I'll go along with it just to humour her.'

Marisa put me into a trance, and asked me to imagine myself sitting in a cinema and seeing my life projected up on a screen in front of me like a film. I could scroll through the film, backwards and forwards, at will. Could I find a moment where food had been a problem? And then something fascinating happened. I was instantly transported back to when I was about nine years old. I was in the kitchen of our old house, stealing money from my mum's purse. Then I hopped onto my bike and cycled two miles away to a sweet shop outside the town – a sweet shop I knew nobody, least of all my parents, would see me in – and I bought a carrier bag full of sweets and chocolate. When I got home again, I went upstairs and hid the bag in my wardrobe – a secret place, where I could hide and eat in private. I remember feeling sad, guilty, ashamed and comforted all at the same time. 'Now find an earlier time,' Marisa said, 'a time when this problem first began. What's happening?' Whoosh. I rewound my film, going through years in just seconds, until I settled on a time when I was just four years old. I was distressed and confused, sitting at the dinner table and crying for my mother. I had woken up that morning to discover that she'd disappeared – rushed off to hospital in the middle of the night. I didn't know then that my mum, pregnant with my little brother, was suffering

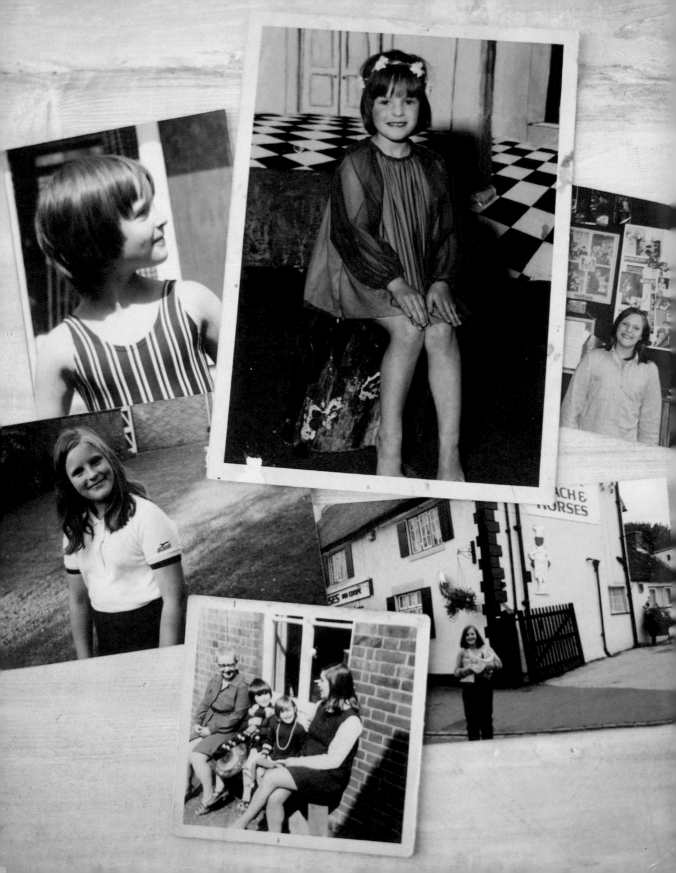

from placenta praevia. My childish mind could only process what was my reality at the time… that I had been abandoned. My mother was ill. Would she die? As it turned out she needed to be hospitalized for over two months. My poor Dad, an unreconstructed 1970s father with a full-time job, was now a single parent. He did the best thing he could think of – feed me up. And boy, did he feed me up! To ease my pain, he showed me love through food. Or more specifically, through adult-sized plates of deep-fried cod, chips, beans and jelly. My mum tells me now that every time we visited her in hospital I would march in, getting plumper by the week, and troop straight over to the washbasin without saying a word to her. Once there, and I remember this vividly, I would wash my hands for an hour and sing, 'Yummy yummy yummy, there's room in my tummy, for some more… for some MORE.' I refused to look at my mother, or speak to her for the whole two months. Freud would have had a field day, I'm sure. But inside, I was a frightened little girl who was disorientated and anxious. I'd learnt Life Lesson Number One to my great cost. When in doubt: EAT.

THE GIFT OF THE PRESENT

You may be wondering what happened after that. Did the hypnotherapy session work? Did I report back that it was a miracle cure for weight loss? Well, actually, yes I did. At the time, I wasn't aware that anything much had happened, other than a rather emotional trip down memory lane. But as the days and weeks passed, I started to behave differently around food precisely as Marisa had predicted I would. I noticed that I was making healthier choices when it came to cooking and eating.

I did a spring clean of my kitchen cupboards and chucked out all the crisps, biscuits, pasta sauces and tins of custard. I replaced sweets with fruit; spaghetti with lentils; and baked beans with fresh veg. I made a note of what I ate, weighed myself regularly and took an interest in my health. People started to notice I was dropping weight. In a matter of weeks, I had lost over two stone. What's interesting to me is that Marisa had asked me during our hypnotherapy session what weight I would like to be. 'Nine stone seven pounds,' I replied. I hit that target to the very last ounce. I road tested eight different diets while I was presenting *Supersize v Superskinny*. The only one that worked for me was hypnotherapy. Not bad for just one session, is it?

Renewed, refreshed, rewired, I was starting to take food more seriously in all aspects of my life. My career as a TV presenter was taking off and I was making a name for myself as the host of popular, prime-time shows about weight loss. I wrote my own diet book, collaborated with experts and became interested in helping other people to change their lives. I was no saint, mind. I still enjoyed a binge on curry or a bottle of red wine and a bag of chocolate – after all, I'm a normal (greedy) woman. But it wasn't until I fronted a new series called *Secret Eaters* for Channel 4 that something really clicked for me. The idea behind the show was that they would secretly film overweight people, using hidden cameras and private investigators, and then confront them back in the TV studio with the 'evidence' of their overeating. Once they'd faced the reality of their ever-expanding waistlines, the team would put them on a healthy-eating plan for several weeks and track their transformation. I should make it clear here that all the contributors had applied to be on the show because they all wanted to lose weight, and simply had no idea what was making them fat. Almost without exception, I could predict who would go on to completely transform their lives. Much depended on the reaction they gave when they saw, for the first time, the hidden-camera footage of themselves eating. Imagine seeing yourself, in private, slumped in front of your TV scoffing a 12-inch pizza in your pyjamas. Maybe you'd do a belch and pick your nose. Maybe your boobs are resting on your belly as you crack open another beer. And that's just the guys. Many people didn't recognize themselves. Some people just laughed and enjoyed the spectacle. But those people who paused, watched in disbelief, and then cried, were more often than not the ones who went on to change. Something shifted for them, something very deep. They were finally exposed, their denial laid bare. They were forced to confront not only what they were eating but what was eating them. This interested me. This interested me very much, particularly given my own experience as a chubby child and an overweight adult. Food is a crutch. Food is a friend. But ultimately, too much food makes us a prisoner of our own self-constructed misery.

It was while I was working on *Secret Eaters* that I met psychologist and diet expert Dr Christy Fergusson. As well as secretly filming overweight people in their everyday lives, the show also put science to the test by doing psychological stunts on the public, to prove just how susceptible we all are to overeating. If we could show how easily we overeat, we could also show how easily we can combat it. Christy was key in helping to prove the research, and it was meeting her, as well as working with the entire team on that brilliant show, that prompted me to take things a little further. After all, I knew loads about this diet stuff right? I'd shifted a ton of weight myself right? Right. But I was still picking at the Jaffa cakes between takes on the studio floor. And I was still a fan of contouring 'shapewear'. Why? Why? Why? I needed to find the final piece of the jigsaw…

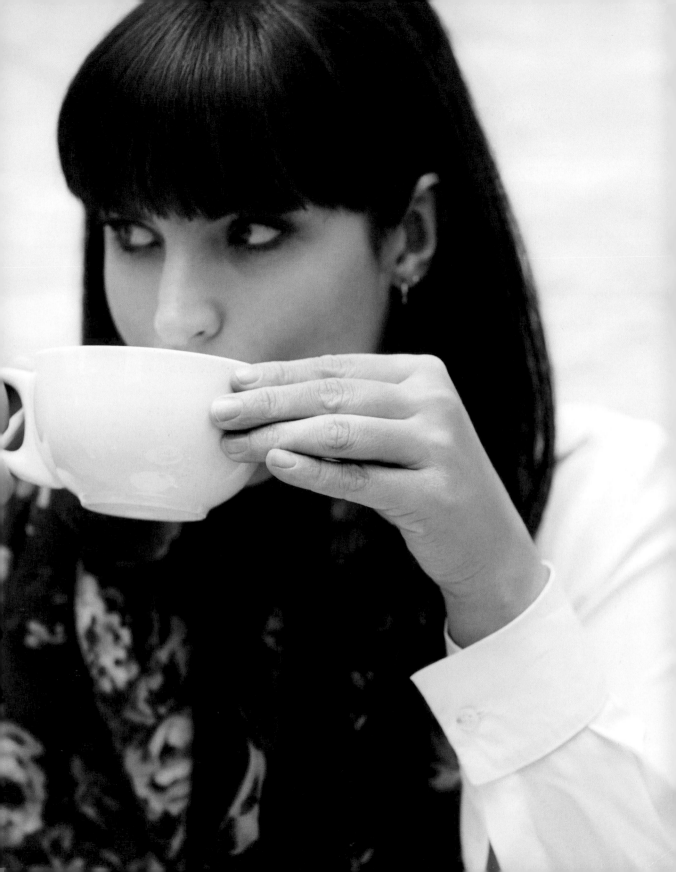

FUTURE PERFECT

So I decided to train as a hypnotherapist myself.

The power of the mind is a magical and mysterious thing. The power of the mind enables us to shape not just our bodies, but our future. The power of the mind is the difference between success… and failure. And the power of the mind is what has urged me to bring all my knowledge and experience into one book – to help you to achieve what you're truly capable of.

Hypnotherapy works. It's a fact. Meeting Marisa Peer changed my life in a surprising and positive way, which is why I asked her to collaborate with me on this book. Her expertise is invaluable in helping us transform ourselves just by using our subconscious mind.

Psychology is what shapes and drives us: fact. And so I also asked Dr Christy Fergusson to collaborate with me on this book. She brings her expert knowledge on the mind to these pages to prove to us that if we want a different life – a different way to eat – then it is merely a thought away.

Our challenge was this: using the power of hypnosis, some practical psychology, plus a healthy-eating plan, would it be possible to drop a dress size without even really trying? We all thought so. So together, we promise to rearrange your mind, as well as rearrange your menu.

'THE POWER OF THE MIND IS A MAGICAL AND MYSTERIOUS THING.'

HOW THIS BOOK WORKS: THE THREE-STEP PROGRAMME

Mind Over Fatter has been designed as a three-step programme using hypnosis, mind management and a healthy-eating plan to totally maximize your weight-loss success.

If you prefer, you may want to focus on just one, or even two, of those steps. For example, if you love the idea of the hypnosis and healthy-eating plan, but aren't interested in the mind management, then OK. The book will still work for you. Likewise, if you just want to follow the recipes, then cool, you'll still feel the health benefits and drop some weight. This book is versatile, deliberately. But to be honest, if you follow all three steps, then the programme is a complete power tool for change.

For many of you, this may well be the first time that you'll find yourselves eating to live – not living to eat. I'm looking to empower each and every one of you to understand yourselves better – to understand your mind-to-mouth behaviour… and to take control.

After all, this isn't so much a diet as a way of living a much healthier, happier life.

Not bad when all you've had to do is think, is it?

SEE
YOURSELF SLIM

This much we know: hypnosis works. It has an impact on the brain that can be measured scientifically. Did you know that the subconscious mind is responsible for 90 per cent of our actions? That's right. You may *think* you're making decisions consciously, but in fact, you're not at all. So it makes sense that if we can talk to the subconscious through hypnosis in order to change its choices then we can change our behaviour too. It's incredibly powerful, effective and safe. To help you do this, this book comes with a link to a free *Mind Over Fatter* Hypnotherapy download (see page 68). In this I'm going to use hypnosis to change the way you relate to food. You will no longer need food as an emotional crutch, addictive pleasure or mindless fuel. Instead, you'll only eat what you need – and make better, healthier choices to boot. *All we ask is that you listen to your download every day, for at least 14 days.* The repetition will help to reinforce the message, so please stick with it. You should start to notice immediate, subtle changes in your behaviour around food. Watch out for them – and smile to yourself when you realize that the difference is already beginning.

THINK
YOURSELF SLIM

While your *unconscious* mind is making subtle changes in behaviour you're not even aware of, Step Two is all about keeping the *conscious* mind busy – focusing on what you can do practically to help your weight loss. The conscious mind is the problem solver. It likes to think, to focus, to plan. In this step, we're going to give you some simple psychological tips that can make a massive difference to your waistline. These aren't just gimmicks; they're scientifically proven fact. Facts that scientists have known for years. Facts that will help you feel more in control of your choices.

★3★

EAT
YOURSELF SLIM

In Step One you've programmed your subconscious mind to work away below decks to change your negative patterns; in Step Two you're using your conscious mind to make better choices around food. You've been given the toolkit and you're already using it. Step Three is the final boost: a simple and nutritious 14-day healthy-eating plan with 60 calorie-conscious recipes that are perfect for the whole family to follow. Of course you can follow it for longer, if you choose, but in 14 days we'd expect to see you starting to drop weight naturally. You should feel leaner, lighter and healthier. The scales and your clothes will tell you that you're on the way to a slimmer you.

IT'S NOT YOUR FAULT YOU'RE FAT . . .

It's a fact. May has been officially named as the month when thousands of women start their 'beach body countdown'. And I count myself as one of those women. One year, in a knee-jerk reaction to stepping on the scales, I found myself signing up to a crazy 'lose seven pounds in seven days' diet plan, gripped by panic about having to squeeze into a bikini in less than six weeks. The thing is, I'm fully aware that crash diets are doomed to failure but that didn't stop me exercising like GI Jane twice a day and eating nothing but sprouts. In the immortal words of Olivia Newton John, 'You'd better shape up' was my mantra. And as she was a woman who had to be *sewn* into those shiny disco slacks, I believe every word she says...

But it was the same the year before, and the year before that, and the year before... you get the picture. So this got me thinking. Are British women trapped in a diet cycle we're not even aware of? Less calorie-controlled and more calendar-controlled?

According to one study, women spend an average of six months a year counting calories in a never-ending quest for the perfect figure. But which six months are we talking about, and does it cause the inevitable, roller-coaster 'yo-yo' weight loss experts warn us against? I think it does. Read on, and let me know if any of this sounds familiar...

NEW YEAR NEW YOU

How many of you started your January New Year's resolution list with: 'Lose some weight' and 'Join the gym'? I speak from experience when I say the average Brit will gain up to 6 pounds over the festive period – with each of us eating around 7,000 calories on Christmas Day *alone*. Given that women need no more than 2,000 calories a day, most of us will have blown that by breakfast. By the time it gets to Twelfth Night we're practically gagging on the Quality Street. It's no accident then that newspapers, magazines and publishers all push their 'new year, new you' diet regimes in our first week back at work.

Curiously though, despite being fatter than at any other time of the year, we also fall off the diet wagon much sooner. January is a miserable month, we know. And what with the post-Christmas credit-card debt, gloomy weather and a return to work and school, no one could blame the 80 per cent of us who throw in the towel on healthy eating after little more than a month.

BEACH BODY COUNTDOWN

It was Oscar Wilde who said, 'I can resist anything except temptation…' and I'm going to add my own wisdom with '… especially if it's covered in chocolate'. I'm talking Easter. And I'm talking eggs. In 2014 80 million Easter eggs were sold in the UK. I know this because I ate most of them. Seventy per cent of us were so mesmerized by those shiny foil gems, we jacked in any attempt at healthy eating for the whole of the Easter period. And a staggering 75 per cent of us have admitted to eating up to four of them over the spring break. This brings us back to May and the 'beach body countdown'. It's the official mid-year panic as women up and down the country realize they have to grease themselves into a Lycra thong and sweat it out on a public beach somewhere, all in the name of 'relaxation'. It's the six-week bikini dash – and ever conscious of our perennial paranoia, the magazines are ready with their quick-fix diets. Nothing tastes as good as the fear of having to stride out naked in public. Nothing.

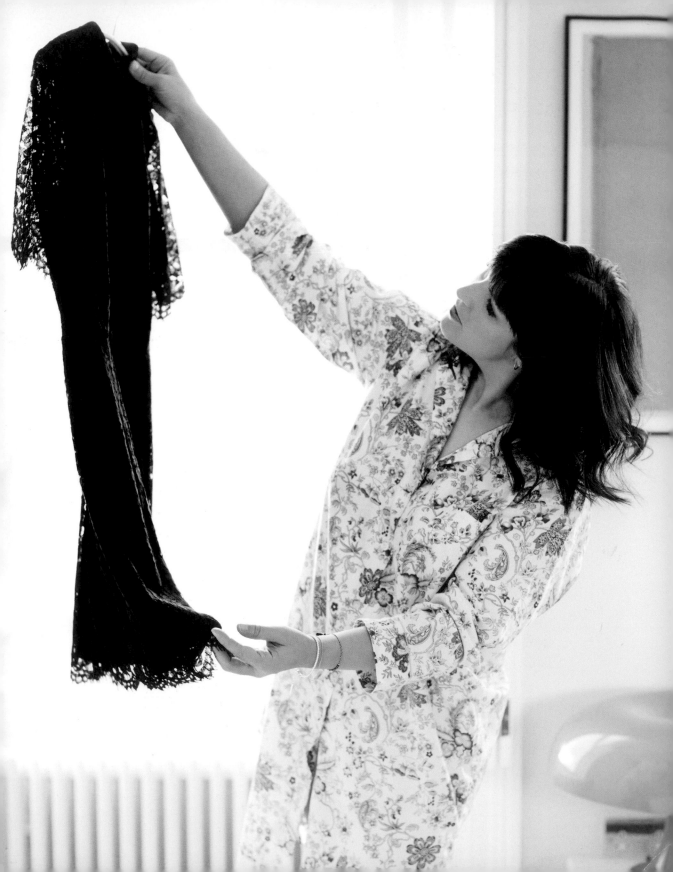

MISTLETOE MARATHON

Autumn. Log fires, leaf-soaked country walks and a diet-girl's best friend – the 60 denier black tight. But what's that you say? Only six weeks until Christmas! You mean I've only got *six weeks* to fit into that little black dress?! And so the mistletoe marathon begins – the race to slim into something so utterly sparkly and *shiny*, it's a miracle we don't all get signed up as extras on *Strictly Come Dancing*. Search online for 'Christmas diet plan' and you get more than 51 million results. Now call me Bad Santa, but why are we all struggling to lose up to a stone only to put it all back on again –and more mind – in just a matter of days? Someone, somewhere, is pulling our Christmas cracker...

CONFUSED?

The trouble is that we're pulled in two different directions. On the one hand we want to feel confident by aspiring to look like the celebrities we're bombarded with in magazines. On the other hand, we're hounded by advertisers' messages telling us that we *deserve* to treat ourselves. Society says 'Eat, drink and be merry' but it also says 'Not too much, fatty'.

The UK diet market is a multi-billion pound industry, yet go into any supermarket and you'll find offers on high-calorie snacks. Our schizophrenic relationship with food is on display in all its glory. It's no wonder we're gluttons for punishment.

So don't beat yourself up any more if you're struggling to lose those extra pounds. In many ways, it really isn't your fault you're fat.

Breaking that co-dependence is not a question of willpower: it's a question of mind power.

DIETS OVER THE DECADES

I read recently that most women have been on more diets than they have had lovers. Diets are nothing new – in fact they've been going for 2,000 years.

Lord Byron, the celebrated Romantic poet who was 'mad, bad and dangerous to know', became something of a diet icon, popularizing his cleanse-and-purge vinegar regime. It was the Victorians, who were so obsessed with the 'aesthetic', that invented the kind of fad diets we're familiar with now. And the trend stuck.

Here are some hungry highlights from more recent decades:

★1900s★
FLETCHERISM AND THE 'CHEW CHEW' CRAZE

American entrepreneur Horace Fletcher's hugely popular weight-loss regime involved chewing food well over a hundred times, and then spitting it out. The idea was that liquid, undigested food could not cause weight gain. He gained the nickname 'The Great Masticator'.

'DIETS ARE NOTHING NEW – IN FACT THEY'VE BEEN GOING FOR 2,000 YEARS.'

★1920s★
CALORIE COUNTING

Lulu Hunt Peters, an American doctor and author, published the first bestselling weight-loss book in 1918, selling two million copies. *Diet and Health: With Key to the Calories* was the first time anyone had highlighted the importance of calories in food. Through her newspaper column 'Diet and Health' she popularized the idea of dieting as self-control, and lost over 50 pounds herself by restricting her intake to 1,200 calories a day.

★1930s★
THE HAY DIET

The Hay Diet, invented by the American physician William Hay following a protracted illness, is one of the most famous food-combining fads. His idea was that all food was either protein, carbohydrate, or neutral. According to his rules, protein and starch should never be eaten in the same meal.

★1950s★
THE CABBAGE SOUP DIET

An extreme fad diet, the Cabbage Soup Diet involved radical weight loss through consuming little more than cabbage soup. Normally a seven-day plan, dieters could supplement the soup with limited fruit, vegetables and meat. What you'd lose in pounds, you'd gain in flatulence.

★1960s★
WEIGHT WATCHERS

Founded in 1963 by overweight American housewife Jean Nidetch, Weight Watchers has grown to become one of the biggest diet brands in the world. Hugely successful, the diet is based on a points system in which the saturated fat and calorie content of foods has already been worked out. Depending on their weight, slimmers are assigned a daily 'points' allowance which they must stick to. It's a simple but clever, calorie-deficit plan.

★1970s★
THE SLIM FAST DIET

The famous meal-replacement plan. The mantra: 'A shake for breakfast, a shake for lunch, then a sensible dinner' became a diet staple. Although the brand has now developed, it originally involved two low-calorie shakes a day and then just one calorie-controlled meal.

★1980s★
THE F-PLAN DIET

The F-Plan Diet, created by British author and founder of *Slimming Magazine*, Audrey Eyton, promoted healthy weight loss by restricting calories to fewer than 1,500 a day, whilst at the same time increasing dietary fibre. *The F-Plan Diet* book subsequently became a top-10 bestseller.

★1990s★
THE ZONE DIET

A diet aimed at keeping insulin and blood sugar levels stable to promote weight loss, the Zone Diet structured calorie-controlled meals into a 40 per cent carbs, 30 per cent protein, 30 per cent fat ratio and became a celebrity-fuelled phenomenon in the nineties.

★2000s★
THE ATKINS DIET

Although first devised in the seventies by US doctor Dr Robert Atkins, the diet truly became an international craze in the noughties with the publication of *Dr Atkins New Diet Revolution*. His principle was to eat very few carbohydrates, but plenty of fat and protein. Although weight loss could be rapid, side effects included bad breath and headaches.

★2010s★
FASTING

Fasting, otherwise known as Intermittent Fasting or the 5:2 Diet, has become the current diet obsession. It involves eating normally for five days of the week, and then restricting food to around 500 calories on the other two days. The idea gained traction in the UK after Dr Michael Mosley investigated the health benefits of fasting in a BBC documentary. He lost weight, improved his health – and a diet sensation was born.

SO WHAT'S EATING YOU?

Most of us can find ourselves overeating sometimes. But for some of us it's a serious problem that can lead to weight gain, obesity and unhappiness. But why? As I discovered when hypnotherapist Marisa Peer regressed me through the film of my life, underlying emotional issues almost always tend to be what make us overeat. And because overeating has an emotional origin, trying to stop it logically will fail. Once we understand and accept this, then we can start to become – and stay – free of it.

When I first met Marisa she told me there are five categories of eaters: addictive, emotional, habitual, ignorant and destructive. Through talking to her I discovered that I'm both an addictive and an emotional eater. When I'm upset or feeling bad about myself I'll punish myself with food that I *know* isn't good for me… but I can't stop. Why would I go and steal money for sweets when I was nine years old and then hide them in my bedroom? Just knowing which type of eater you are can be a lightbulb moment. Now I know, I'm able to take control of how I eat. So, what's eating you? Once you know the answer, you'll be one step closer to fixing it.

IDENTIFY YOUR TRIGGERS

There's so much going on behind our unconscious eating habits. But it's hard to fix what you don't understand. So before we start, try answering the questions on the following pages to see which type of eater you are… and what will help you to break free. Answer every question for each type of eater. If you answer yes to more than half the questions on each page you can identify yourself with that category. And once you know your emotional triggers… you have the power to change.

★ 1 ★

ADDICTIVE EATERS

★ Do you think about food all day?

★ Do you eat really fast so you don't fully experience your
food and then want more?

★ Do you repeat this pattern over and over?

★ Do you crave sugar?

★ If you have sugary snacks in the house are you unable
to resist them until they are all gone?

★ Do you eat sensibly all day but lose control in the evenings?

★ Are there foods – packets of biscuits, sharing-size bags of
crisps, family-size chocolate bars – that once you start eating
you can't stop?

★ Do you eat the food you're craving so fast you didn't enjoy it…
or even taste it?

If you have answered 'yes' to more than half the questions,
you are an addictive eater.

·2·

EMOTIONAL EATERS

★ Do you use food to block out feelings of loneliness, unhappiness or boredom?

★ Do you eat when you feel under pressure?

★ Do you prefer to eat alone?

★ Do you eat differently when you're eating with others?

★ Do you eat in secret?

★ Do you find it hard to be without chocolate, sweets and biscuits?

★ Do you particularly crave carbohydrates when you are unhappy?

★ Do you believe that certain foods comfort you and make you feel better?

★ Do you eat something after an argument or if you feel tense or wound up because it changes your state of mind?

If you have answered 'yes' to more than half the questions, you are an emotional eater.

∗3∗

HABITUAL EATERS

★ Do you eat quickly and finish before others?

★ Do you finish everything and always clear your plate?

★ Do you no longer recognize when you are full and when you are hungry?

★ Do you eat whenever food is in front of you, regardless of whether or not you are hungry?

★ Do you put on weight predominantly around your stomach?

★ Do you find it hard to throw food away or 'waste' it?

★ Do you remember always being made to finish meals as a child?

★ Do you use every occasion – watching TV, on a train, at the cinema – to eat?

★ Do you have an overweight partner or children?

If you have answered 'yes' to more than half the questions, you are an habitual eater.

★4★
IGNORANT EATERS

★ Do you think that all salad is healthy including coleslaw and the dressing?

★ Do you think pizza is a complete meal because it has some peppers and tomatoes on it?

★ Do you eat a lot of bread, pasta, potatoes, cereal, milk and cheese?

★ Do you believe all foods labelled low fat, reduced sugar and diet must be good for you?

★ Do you count potatoes as vegetables?

★ Do you think fruit bars, fruit drinks and canned fruit are as good as fresh fruit?

★ Do you think all fruit is healthy so you can eat as much as you like and still lose weight?

★ Do you think you have to eat before you exercise or you won't have enough energy?

★ Do you struggle to understand what calories are and how many you need each day?

If you have answered 'yes' to more than half the questions, you are an ignorant eater.

★5★

DESTRUCTIVE EATERS

★ Do you feel anxious and uncomfortable when you are slimmer?

★ Do you still buy clothes in a larger size and keep the clothes from when you were bigger?

★ Do you lose the same 10 pounds (or thereabouts) every year only to gain it back?

★ Do you feel more comfortable in winter – when your body is covered up – than in summer, when you have to wear less?

★ Do you sabotage your diet every time you come close to your ideal weight?

★ Do you celebrate your weight loss success by resuming eating the foods you had denied yourself?

★ Do you find that as a beach holiday approaches you start to sabotage your diet and then spend the holiday avoiding the beach and trying out lots of restaurants instead?

★ Do you fear being attractive so much that when you're asked on a date, you begin to overeat as the date gets nearer?

If you have answered 'yes' to more than half the questions, you are a destructive eater.

UNDERSTANDING YOUR TYPE

As you work out which category of eater you are it's normal
to fit into more than one type. I fit into two and it totally makes
sense. Broadly speaking, 75 per cent of us are emotional eaters
or addictive eaters; 20 per cent are habitual or ignorant eaters;
and only around 5 per cent fall into the destructive category.
Nearly half of us use food to alter our mood every day.

★ ★ ★
ADDICTIVE EATERS
★ ★ ★

Addictive eaters crave sugar, caffeine, junk food, fizzy drinks
and refined carbohydrates. They are literally addicted to these
foods. They can't resist them. They eat them really quickly.
They can't just eat a little of them, and eating these foods just
makes them want more. Crisps, chocolate, biscuits, sweets and
fast food contain a cocktail of chemical additivies such as
colourings, trans fats and preservatives as well as naturally
occuring ingredients such as salt and sugar, which can be highly
addictive. These chemicals make the brain release the 'feel
good' neurotransmitter dopamine in the same way drugs do.
Over the years eating these foods can become a substitute for
happiness and will lead bingers to become addicted. And like
all addicts they need more and more of the dopamine just
to get the same effect.

*So what can you do about it? Like all addictions the only cure is to stop
altogether. You don't have to live on mung beans and bean sprouts –*

there's a world of healthy alternatives out there that aren't full of addictive chemicals. And once you give your body better and more natural food you will forget about junk very quickly, often within 14 days. If you stop feeding the addiction it will, eventually, just go away. Once it has, you'll find that you'll be able to control yourself around these unhealthy foods without reverting back to old patterns.

★ ★ ★
EMOTIONAL EATERS
★ ★ ★

Emotional eaters try to get rid of a bad feeling fast and try to feel good even faster by eating refined carbohydrates – 'comfort foods' – and often in bulk. They eat lots of toast or a big bowl of pasta or cereal and then feel almost sedated. Refined carbohydrates fill us up quickly – we feel satisfied and 'calm' – but it never lasts. It's no coincidence that, in decades gone by, patients with mental disorders were given lots of carbohydrate foods because of the calming effect they have. Think about it, when we're low we're often drawn to sugary foods. Comfort can be found – briefly – in soft, sweet foods, like ice cream, chocolate or cake, which remind us of childhood. As a child, your needs may have been met with sugar… but as an adult, this will never be the case.

The quickest way to stop this is to recognize what you're doing and break the vicious cycle. Stop using carbohydrates as medication. Instead try a hot drink, or a bowl of warm vegetable soup. Hot liquids are comforting and don't put pressure on your digestion, or cause stress in your body, the way excess carbohydrates do.

★ ★ ★

HABITUAL EATERS

★ ★ ★

Habitual eaters have usually been brought up to eat everything on their plate. As children, they were conditioned to eat anything to such an extent that they continue this way of eating purely out of habit. They will eat at every occasion and eat everything in front of them without being aware of whether they're hungry or not… or even if they like the food or not. They hate to waste food and will never throw it away.

Just being aware that you acquired these habits, most likely through childhood, will help you to get back the ability to leave food when you're full. See leaving food as empowering. Try returning food to the fridge for another day, giving it to someone else or taking it home in a doggy bag if you're in a restaurant. You don't have to eat it just because it's there. The more you practise leaving a little something, the sooner you can escape your childhood conditioning.

★ ★ ★

IGNORANT EATERS

★ ★ ★

Ignorant eaters have been completely brainwashed by food manufacturers to believe that what they are eating is healthy or harmless. They might eat a lot of convenience foods and ready meals and believe they're as good as home-cooked food; they might exist primarily on diet foods and drinks but still have a weight problem. They tend to eat a lot of refined carbohydrate foods believing them to be low-fat and healthy. In fact, the opposite is true – excess carbohydrates raise your insulin levels and keep your body in a constant state of fat storage. Your body isn't aware if you're eating bread, pasta or cake – it converts all carbohydrate into sugar.

So how can you move from being an overweight, ignorant eater, into a slim, informed eater? Make sure you read and understand food labels. Try eating homemade, healthy meals rather than ready-made ones. And definitely start by trying my healthy-eating plan and recipes at the end of the book.

★ ★ ★

DESTRUCTIVE EATERS

★ ★ ★

Destructive eaters sometimes have a deep-rooted need to hide and disguise their sexuality or attractiveness, and often feel vulnerable when they look attractive or desirable. People who have never had enough love often compensate by having more than enough food. This can often be the case when restrictions or controls were put on food – or certain types of food – in their childhood. They like to have big portions, frequent meals and snacks; and always fear they may not get enough. They often feel panicky in a situation where food is shared, in case they get less than other people or don't have enough to feel full. They prefer to dish out their own portions to make absolutely sure they're getting enough.

If this sounds like you, you need to understand that your subconscious mind is the 'feeling' mind – and it still feels you might not get enough. Remind yourself that you are in charge of what, when and how much you eat. You will always have enough food; food will always be there. As you remind yourself of this, the panic response around food will begin to lessen and go.

★ ★ ★

Once you know what type of eater you are, use our free *Mind Over Fatter* Timeline Regression download (see page 40) to work out where your issue with food first started, and why. When you can see this trigger you can start to understand how overeating isn't your fault. You couldn't stop it happening… but you can stop it continuing. And that's where the second download comes in. By using the *Mind Over Fatter* Hypnotherapy download in Step One (see page 68) we'll help you overcome these demons forever.

★ ★ ★

'ONCE YOU CAN SEE THIS TRIGGER YOU CAN START TO UNDERSTAND HOW OVEREATING ISN'T YOUR FAULT.'

FOOD IS THE DRUG

According to new research, due to be published in the United States, a diet of burgers, crisps, sweets and cake will programme your brain into craving even more foods that are high in sugar, salt and fat.

Neuroscientist Dr Paul Kenny carried out the research, which shows how dangerous high sugar foods and artificial foods can be to our health. 'You lose control. It's the hallmark of addiction,' he said. The researchers believe that this is one of the first studies to suggest our brains may react in the same way to junk food as they do to drugs. 'This is the most complete evidence to date that suggests obesity and drug addiction have common neuro-biological foundations,' said Paul Johnson, Dr Kenny's work colleague.

Dr Kenny, who began his research at Guy's Hospital, London, but now works at Florida's Scripps Research Institute, divided rats into three groups for his study.

One group got normal amounts of healthy food to eat. The second group was given restricted amounts of junk food. The last group was given unlimited amounts of junk food, including cheesecake, cheap sponge cakes and chocolate snacks. There were no adverse effects on the first two groups, but the rats who ate as much junk food as they wanted quickly gained weight and started bingeing.

When researchers electronically stimulated the part of the brain that feels pleasure, they found that the rats on unlimited junk food needed more and more stimulation to register the same level of pleasure as the rats on healthier diets. Still fancy that pizza and pud now?

THE MIND OVER FATTER
TIMELINE REGRESSION DOWNLOAD

We're all born with a normal relationship with food: that's why babies don't overeat, don't bolt their food and have no problem leaving food regardless of how delicious it is. So if we accept the premise that we were born with a completely normal attitude to food, it means that somewhere along the line we must have developed an *abnormal* relationship with food. It partly explains why millions of us now struggle with our weight.

In our unique *Mind Over Fatter* Timeline Regression download I'm going to help you track back to where, how and why that happened. Once you've pinpointed the origin of your problem, you'll be so much better equipped to fix it. Sometimes, this can be a light bulb moment – it certainly was for me.

Remember I told you that in my timeline I went back to when I was four years old and my mother had been rushed to hospital. I was a confused and frightened little girl unable to understand why she wasn't with me. My dad, not knowing how to cope with my sadness and trying to show me love, filled me up with huge plates of food. The message I learned was that food comforts sadness. The pattern was set, and I spent the next three decades abusing food whenever I was sad or lonely. But once I came to understand this through hypnosis, I was able to change it.

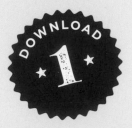

★ ★ ★

HOW WILL IT WORK?

★ ★ ★

★ Go to www.mindoverfatterdownload.co.uk and follow the instructions for the Timeline Regression download.

★ Find a time when you're on your own, and you can relax. Listen to my voice, and just be guided by the words. Your subconscious mind will do the rest.

★ Once you've come out of the trance, make a note of any thoughts, images or memories that came to you. They're important.

★ Once you have the information and you've written it down, practise saying to yourself on a regular basis: 'I know now that my problem stemmed from... and I don't need to do that any more. I choose a healthier me.'

★ You may find that more thoughts and more memories come up over the next few days. That's normal. Just note what they are and add them to your new resolve to move on from the relationship you used to have with food, and to eat in a healthier way from now on.

★ ★ ★

GET READY TO CHANGE . . . YOURSELF

Here's a question for you: what's the link between 62 per cent of adults in the UK being overweight and our diet industry being worth £2 billion? Denial. It's a dirty word, I know, and a grubby little secret shared by all of us in one form or another. Denial is the reason the Channel 4 surveillance series *Secret Eaters* I presented was watched by millions of people. And also why it had one of the most successful weight-loss results of any diet show on TV. It's only when we're faced with the reality of what we're truly eating that we're shocked into action. One of my favourite characters on the series was a chap who'd paid thousands of pounds to have a gastric band fitted only to make it his personal mission to try and cheat it. He'd eat exactly the same amount of food as he did before the operation – just blended. None of us want to believe we eat as much as we really do. And that's one of the reasons we have an obesity epidemic in the western world.

I certainly suffer my fair share of the D word. When I was much heavier, a few years ago, I tried a designer dress on in Selfridges. I was shopping for a big TV event and it was important to me that I looked as glamorous as possible. I've got to tell you, this dress was beautiful. Expensive, sculpted and – on the right person – an object of wonder. I literally spooned my body into this thing. With my face the colour of a double-decker and with a proper sweat on, I shuffled out of the changing room. 'What do you think?' I asked the skinny assistant. With a heart-stopping beat, she said, 'Darling. I say this for your own good. You need to lose at least ten pounds before you can wear a dress like this.

You're a young woman. You've let yourself go. Go on a diet, then come back and see me. I'll make you look fabulous.'

Yes, I was humiliated. Yes, I cried when I got home. And yes… I went on that diet. Denial may well be a powerful force but not as powerful as determination. I went on to lose my excess weight – and I also went on to do a photo shoot in LA in one of the *tightest, weeniest,* drop-dead *gorgeous* dresses out there. I'm never going to be a naturally thin girl – but I can be the best 'me'. Check out the smile on my face – it beats all the tears I've ever shed for not feeling good enough.

Part of the success of any healthy-eating plan is organization. There's a lot of truth in the maxim 'failing to plan is planning to fail'. So with that in mind, here are some of my tried-and-tested tips to boost your chances of successful weight loss. So get ready to change… yourself.

WEIGHTS AND MEASURES

There are myriad diet plans out there that advise you not to weigh or measure yourself – just to go with the flow of your belt buckle and hope for the best. For me, this is all part of what we talked about earlier – denial. How can you possibly gauge your progress if you don't really know what size and weight you were in the first place? For years, when I used to be a member of various slimming clubs, I had a weekly pact with the woman weighing me at the meetings *not* to reveal my weight to me – only to let me know if I'd lost any. I simply couldn't face it. It was only when I was forced to step on the scales for the TV series *Supersize v Superskinny* that I was confronted with the reality of my weight issue. My shock was real and heartfelt. So what I ask of you is this.

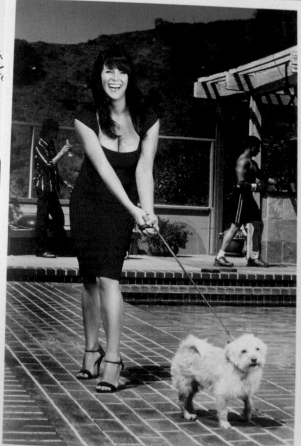

Books (left to right, spines):

ANGELA CARTER — *Nights at the Cir...*

NIALL WILLIAMS — *Four L...*

Jeanette Wint...

EDITH W...

SMITH I Ca...

★ Buy some scales. Place them on a hard surface – the bathroom floor is ideal – and get on them. Take a deep breath, look down and take a note of your weight.

★ Get a tape measure. Measure your waist, hips, bust, thigh and upper arm. Make a note of each number.

★ The good news is you're going to start to see these numbers going down. Repeat the process every week until you're happy with your size.

TAKE BEFORE-AND-AFTER PHOTOS

This works. It really, really works. Earlier this year, I decided to do a test – would it be possible for me to lose weight and see a visible difference in my body after just seven days of careful eating and moderate exercise?

Take a look at my set of photos on the next page. That's after just seven days. It's not dramatic, but it was around a 5-pound weight loss and several inches off the tape measure. Imagine what the improvement could be after a month. So before you begin the plan…

★ Stand in front of a mirror. Take a photo of yourself (naked or in underwear). Save it.

★ Take another at the end of the plan. It could be in two weeks – or a month. Up to you. Place your photos side-by-side so you can judge the difference (there are tons of apps available that enable you to do this).

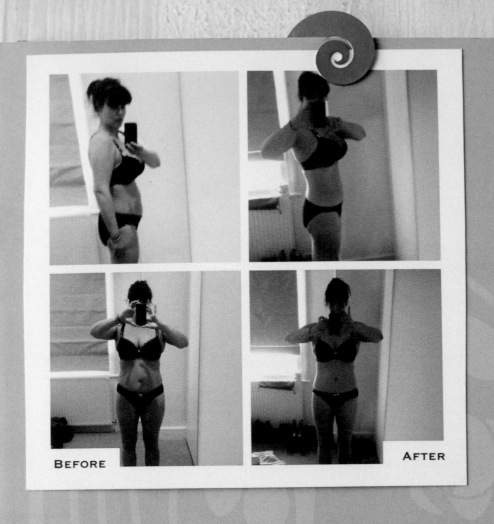

BEFORE   AFTER

THE POWER OF POSITIVE

Here's a thing. I could look at those photos of me and think, 'Gah… I'm so chubby! When am I going to be thin/athletic/ amazing?' etc. and beat myself up for not being perfect. But I'm not going to. Instead, I can look at myself and say, 'I'm not fat. I have a sexy, curvy body. But I enjoy being slimmer. I feel happier when I'm lighter. And I know exactly what to do.'

The fact is that having a positive image of yourself is one of the secrets to successful weight loss. Recently, the cereal brand Special K conducted a survey into how positive thinking can affect the outcome of a diet. A massive 71 per cent of women in their study used the negative term 'fat' to describe themselves, whilst a mere 34 per cent of them start a diet actually believing they'll lose any weight at all. Your subconscious is always listening. By talking to ourselves in a negative way, by denying responsibility for our behaviour and creating a belief system that presupposes defeat, we set ourselves up to fail.

So, go back to the mirror. Stand naked in front of it. Resist the urge to criticize your body. Instead, take a long, hard look from all angles and notice what you like about yourself. Is your body strong? Do you have a great waist maybe? Perhaps your body has performed a miracle like giving birth. Everybody has something good they can say about themselves physically. Focus on it… and encourage yourself to improve and be the best possible you.

KEEP A DIET DIARY

If I had just one tip to help guarantee weight loss, it would be this: keep a diet journal. Several studies have shown that people who keep food diaries are more likely to be successful in losing weight and keeping it off. The simple act of writing down what you've eaten every day instantly increases your awareness of how much you're actually consuming. Instead of mindless grazing you become mindful of your menu.

Keeping a daily journal can also help you identify any negative habits or stumbling blocks you've been previously unaware of. Many people underestimate the calories present in drinks, for example. If they don't 'eat' it, they don't count it. Mistake. Other people skip breakfast and lunch, and then carb load at the end of the day – often consuming far more calories than if they'd spread their meals sensibly. Do you eat when you're stressed, tired or bored? Look at your patterns. Notice what needs to change.

It's entirely up to you what format you choose for your diary. It could be a special book that you like to write in every day – or it could be on your computer or via an app. Regularly add your weight, your measurements, and your before-and-after photos too. Track your transformation. You are your own project.

'INSTEAD OF MINDLESS GRAZING
YOU BECOME MINDFUL
OF YOUR MENU.'

tea break   peppermint tea
and some carrot sticks +

Dinner. pre plan? ... plans? Maybe stir fry

DO YOU SEE IT, HEAR IT, FEEL IT OR THINK IT?

If you are your own project, then knowing yourself and how you tend to process information is going to help make that project a success.

The brain receives around 11 million pieces of information through our senses every second of every day. From the moment that information is received it has to be managed and made sense of. In processing that mass of information, each of us tends to filter it through a favoured sense at any given time. According to Neuro Linguistic Programming (NLP) this is referred to as our Preferred Representational System – those systems being Visual, Auditory, Kinaesthetic and Auditory Digital. Before this gets too heavy, try this out:

Sit somewhere quiet and remember one of your favourite holidays. Try to picture it in your head. What does the scene look like? Can you picture it? What are the sounds around you? How does it feel? Can you remember your journey there?

When you walked into your workplace today what was the first thing you noticed? Was it the decor of the room? The sounds around you? What was the temperature like?

Your answers to these questions should start to help you to work out whether your Preferred Representational System is Visual, Auditory, Kinaesthetic or Auditory Digital. I've created a brief sketch of each type of person below and made suggestions of techniques that might particularly work for you. Of course, this is just a brief snapshot of Representational Systems and how they work. Although some people tend to have a dominant sense, you may also find that you can identify with all of them equally. That's fine. Just take whatever tips you find useful and apply them to 'project me'. You might be surprised by how effective they are.

★ ★ ★

PEOPLE WHO ARE VISUAL:

★ ★ ★

★ Notice how things *look*.

★ Notice decor, scenery, colours, what people are wearing.

★ Can 'picture' things in their mind very clearly.

★ Use language like: 'I see what you mean', 'We don't really see eye-to-eye'.

If this seems like you, it would make sense to make a mood board of how you might like to look. Attach photos of yourself when you were looking your best and rip inspirational pictures out of magazines to focus on. Your before-and-after photos will be really important to you.

★ ★ ★

PEOPLE WHO ARE AUDITORY:

★ ★ ★

★ Notice how things *sound*.

★ Love music, tone and pitch, and can remember verbatim conversations and arguments.

★ Need to 'hear' their thoughts, so tend to speak uninterrupted and at length, in order to process what they think.

★ May not enjoy silence much – instead preferring to have the radio or TV on constantly for company.

★ Use language like: 'I hear what you're saying', 'I'm all ears'.

If this sounds like you, you may want to record some inspirational messages of support from friends or family to listen to, particularly if you hit a stumbling block with your diet. Perhaps there are some motivational downloads you could use, or pieces of music that will energize you.

PEOPLE WHO ARE KINAESTHETIC:

★ Notice how things *feel*.
★ Are sensitive to the physical conditions around them: how comfortable they are in a chair, the temperature of a room.
★ Are aware of their own emotions and, often, the emotions of others around them.
★ Use language like: 'He makes me feel really comfortable', 'I'm having difficulty getting hold of her'.

If that feels like you, you are going to love, love, love the physical sensation of becoming slimmer and lighter. You'll enjoy how your clothes begin to fit better, and the feeling you get when people compliment you on how well you're looking.

PEOPLE WHO ARE AUDITORY DIGITAL:

★ Notice *detail and process*.
★ Like the logical process of things.
★ Think by talking to themselves in their heads and sometimes have difficulty 'switching off'.
★ Prefer to think about how they feel, rather than actually feel it so may come across as unemotional or detached.
★ Use language like: 'It makes total sense to me', 'I understand what you're saying'.

If you think that's you, you'll enjoy recording every detail of your journey – your meals, weight, measurements. You'll want to understand how the hypnosis process works and once you've bought into the facts there'll be no stopping you.

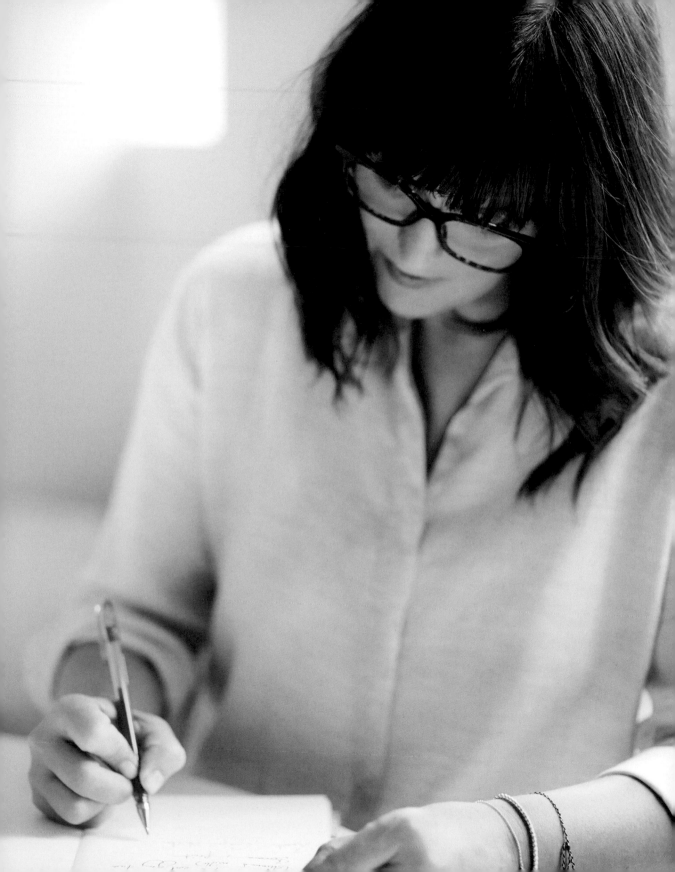

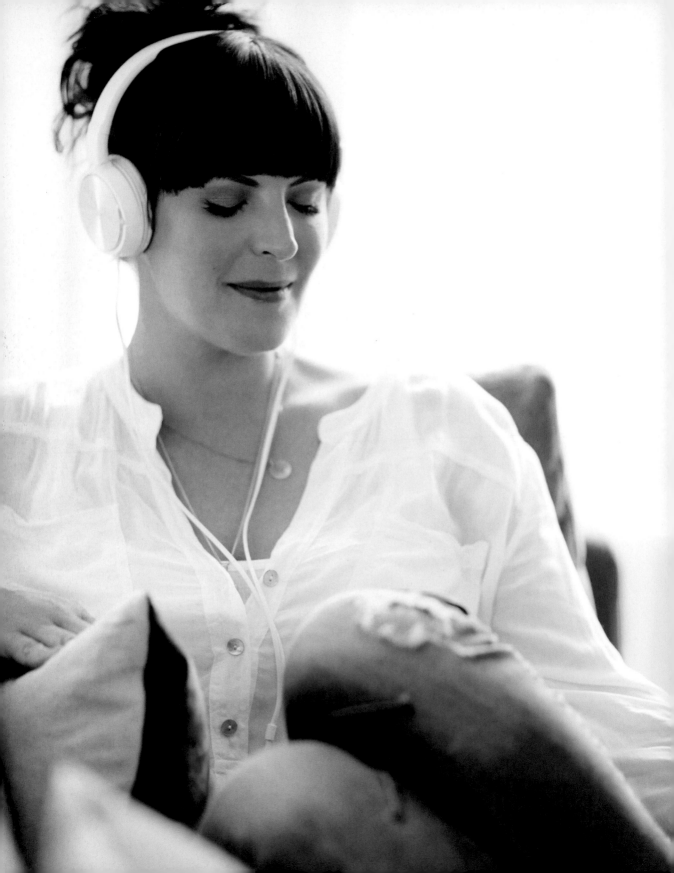

SEE
YOURSELF SLIM

THE POWER OF THE SUBCONSCIOUS MIND

We're born into this world with the most amazing brain. More powerful than any computer known to man, it's capable of doing so much, achieving things beyond the realms of imagination. And yet there are no instructions out there to tell us how to get the best from ourselves. There's no manual that shows us how to programme ourselves for success. So is it any wonder that, despite our amazing brain, we can still get things so badly wrong?

You don't need to have a degree to understand how the mind works when it comes to overeating, eating badly and destructive behaviour. But it does help to know the basics. So I'm going to show you how to understand your mind – and use its power through our free *Mind Over Fatter* Hypnotherapy download – to master your own weight-loss success.

How many times have you heard someone say, 'I'm in two minds about this' or 'Part of me wants to do X, but the other part of me wants to do Y'? That's because your 'mind' actually comprises two parts: your *conscious* mind and your *subconscious* mind. And it's the subconscious mind we're going to be focusing on in this chapter, because it is very, very powerful...

YOUR SUBCONSCIOUS MIND:

Is your emotional, intuitive, creative brain

★

Is responsible for 90 per cent of your actions

★

Is aware of up to 11 million bits of
information at any one moment

★

Is in charge of your habits, behaviour and addictions

★ ★ ★

If that sounds a bit far-fetched, then consider this. How many times have you driven your car, chatting to your mates along the way, and then arrived at your destination with no real memory of the journey there? It just 'happened'. You knew how to get there without looking at a map. You knew how to drive the car without thinking. And you were capable of driving, talking, and maybe listening to the radio all at the same time. *That's* your subconscious taking over. It's on automatic pilot. Studies have shown that our brains begin to prepare for action a fraction of a second before we consciously decide to act. So even if you *think* you're in control of your thoughts, actions and behaviours it's actually your subconscious that's controlling you.

Or what about this? Have you ever had a conversation with someone, maybe in a job interview or on a date, and despite the other person saying all the right things you just don't believe them? Something inside you – your gut instinct – tells you something is wrong. This is really no surprise at all. Only

7 per cent of meaning comes from the words we speak; 38 per cent is taken from tone of voice; and 55 per cent from our body language. So that 'gut instinct' is our subconscious interpreting the subliminal signs, and warning us.

Your wonderful subconscious mind is there to protect you. And it'll do whatever it can to make sure you're safe and happy. The irony is that, in protecting you, it can sometimes confuse destructive behaviour with a positive outcome. Why else would we sink a bottle of wine when we feel stressed? Because the mind links alcohol with relaxation. Smoke cigarettes even though we know they kill? Because we associate cigarettes with good times. Or eat chocolate when we're down? Because chocolate equals comfort.

So let's help the subconscious mind to do its job even better.

'YOUR WONDERFUL SUBCONSCIOUS MIND IS THERE TO PROTECT YOU. AND IT'LL DO WHATEVER IT CAN TO MAKE SURE YOU'RE SAFE AND HAPPY.'

VISUALIZATION EXERCISE

★ Find a time when you can be on your own, and quiet.

★ Create an image in your head of how you'd ideally like to look – and hold that image in your mind.

★ Relax into the image. As well as seeing yourself at your best weight, imagine what it *feels* like to be that way. Your subconscious is your emotional mind and will link that positive feeling with being slim.

Keep re-running the picture so your mind accepts it. You will be programming your subconscious to begin to make changes in your behaviour to help you reach the goal weight you are visualizing.

★ ★ ★

MAKE A MOOD BOARD

★ ★ ★

To help you focus on seeing yourself as slim, make a mood board. Put it somewhere you'll see it every day. Stick on pictures of you when you were slimmer to remind you that if you were like that once, you can be like that again. Add images of things that inspire you: other people you admire; clothes you'd like to wear; activities you'd like to do; or healthy food you'd like to cook. Doing this will begin to train your mind into seeing you as slimmer and accepting you acting the way a slimmer person acts.

The more you visualize, the more you will believe your goal is possible. Very successful people visualize all the time. We can all change our thinking and the mental pictures we make, and as we improve them, we improve everything. Remember… we get the outcome we expect.

SEE THINGS DIFFERENTLY

In order to be slim you must first be able to see yourself as slim. And I know myself that's not easy if you haven't seen yourself as a slim person for many, many years. But when we stand in front of the mirror and think, 'I can't lose weight' or ' I'll never be slim in a million years' we make it impossible for anything else to be true. We're creating an image that we eventually become. Why? Because the strongest, most powerful force in the subconscious mind is the need to remain consistent with how we define ourselves. In that sense, you get the outcome you expect, or (and we've all experienced this) you create a self-fulfilling prophecy. The subconscious mind believes whatever you tell it. So if you tell it diets don't work or you hate exercise then – you guessed it – your diet won't work and you'll never go to the gym. So it's time to change how you see yourself.

Your ability to imagine yourself as slimmer sends a powerful message to your subconscious mind that *this* is the outcome you really desire. Remember, your subconscious wants to protect you – so it'll start to find new ways to help you achieve your goal of a healthier, slimmer you if you truly believe that's what you want. Your mind always influences your body – so start believing what you tell it, and quit the negative talk.

A BIT OF STRAIGHT-TALKING

Your subconscious mind does what it believes you want it to do. So you need to make sure it's getting the right message. When you are specific, and communicate with it using clear, positive words then any misinterpretation is less likely to happen. Tell it what you really desire using direct commands and images. For example: 'I want to be a size 10'; 'I want to look great in a bikini'; 'I want to make healthier choices'; 'I want to enjoy exercise'. Tell it repeatedly. This ensures that your mind clearly and emphatically understands what it is that you need. Before I went under hypnosis with Marisa Peer, she asked me what weight I would like to be. 'Nine and a half stone,' I told her. I hit that target to the ounce – my subconscious was listening.

The way you feel about any situation is linked to two things: the pictures you make in your head and the words you say to yourself. If you use words like: 'I *love* pasta!' or 'I *cannot* live without my chocolate' then that's how your mind will respond to these foods. But if you look at a plate of pasta and think: 'Hmmm, stodgy, white glue that makes me bloat' then your subconscious mind will respond to that instead. Say to yourself: 'I'm choosing to eat fruit instead of dessert. I'm choosing to feel great about that because I have chosen to be slimmer'. It's a clear instruction to your mind.

Your mind has no ability to disagree with what you tell it, so you'll do better when you tell yourself positive things. And don't just tell it occasionally – tell it all the time.

KICKING THE HABIT

Your mind loves, and will always return to, what is familiar. So to change any habit you have to make the familiar unfamiliar, and the unfamiliar familiar. That's a tongue-twister! Is lounging around on the sofa eating packets of crisps familiar? Does it feel unfamiliar to go outside and walk? If walking outside becomes a regular habit then it will become familiar, and lounging around covered in crisp crumbs will become unfamiliar. If you have tea with full-fat milk and two sugars, that is familiar. Tea with skimmed milk and no sugar will seem unfamiliar. But stick with it – you'll be amazed how soon it becomes a habit and you'll even find the old way tastes horrible.

Once an idea has been accepted by the mind, it tends to remain. The longer it is held, the more likely it is to become a fixed way of thinking. It's how habits of action are formed – both good and bad. First is the habit of thought: 'I need that chocolate to get through the afternoon'. And then the habit of action: eating the chocolate even though we don't need it and swore we would resist it. We have habits of thinking as well as habits of action, but the thought always comes first. So if we want to change our actions, we must begin by changing our thoughts. We all have the power to make good habits a part of our life, and bad habits history. If only it were that simple, though. Those fixed habits are fixed in the subconscious, and however much the conscious mind wants to change them, it's going to find it hard.

PAIN AND PLEASURE

Part of the job of your subconscious mind is to move you towards pleasure, and away from pain. It wants to protect you at all costs. So as long as you believe that whatever destructive behaviour you're repeating makes you happy and helps you to cope, then your subconscious will link that behaviour to pleasure and repeat it ad nauseum. But you *can* choose what to link pain and pleasure to, and so change the pattern.

People who successfully lose weight and keep it off tend to

have a very clear definition that being slim is 'pleasure' and worth working for, whereas eating destructively is 'pain' and should be avoided. Try it. Can you link pleasure to looking great and being healthy instead? Remind yourself that eating healthy food in the right amounts is a better reward for your body than pigging out on crisps and chocolate. Making the right choices and changing your beliefs will make you more successful at permanent weight loss.

CLEAR OUT THE COBWEBS

Strong emotion makes us stupid. We can quite literally get 'hijacked' by feelings and then repeat the same negative behaviour again and again. How often have you been gripped by anger, grief, jealousy or guilt, said or done something you've regretted and then thought, 'Why did I *do* that? I didn't really mean it.'

The reason we do it is because the subconscious mind is the emotional, feeling mind. And when it is in thrall to strong emotion it will automatically act on old, outdated beliefs – beliefs that were often formed in childhood. And when you distil those beliefs down, they tend to reveal the same picture in all of us... the fear that we're not loved; not good enough; or don't deserve to be happy.

When I was nine, I was an anxious little girl who stole money for sweets because I found comfort in secretly eating. For years, my subconscious mind linked overeating to coping with pain. Until I recognized the pattern, and changed it. If you've listened to your Timeline Regression download (see page 40), then you may well have pinpointed where your own problems with food first started. It's time to clear out those cobwebs. Understanding how your subconscious mind works will help you to let go of those thoughts, beliefs and behaviours, which you grew out of years ago.

WORK IT

Once a new suggestion has been accepted by the subconscious mind, it becomes easier for additional suggestions to be accepted. That's why you can so often get on a roll with dieting. Suddenly you're eating differently, exercising, taking your own food to work and shunning cakes. It all fits into place because you're giving yourself better suggestions and your mind is acting on them. But it's important when you're giving your mind new suggestions that you keep working at it. See your subconscious as a muscle. Use it differently and it will work differently. But you can't just use that muscle once and expect it to be bigger and stronger. One session of exercise isn't going to be enough – you have to continue it. The good news is that the more you use your mind differently the easier it becomes. Soon it stops being what you do – and becomes a part of who you are.

WILL AND POWER VERSUS WILLPOWER

I've seen people be really hard on themselves because they believe they don't have the 'willpower' to make positive changes in their lives. The fact is willpower is not enough to help you lose weight. Willpower is a conscious demand – and the subconscious mind can make the conscious mind do *whatever* it wants. That's why when you subconsciously believe that eating a bag of crisps will cheer you up, but you consciously want to resist them, the subconscious almost always wins. Making a *conscious* effort to resist those crisps is pointless if the subconscious mind believes something totally different.

Your conscious mind has a will. But it's the subconscious mind that has the power. And while the conscious mind requires effort, the subconscious mind is effortless. Remember how learning to drive a car for the first time took effort? You had to use your conscious mind. But in time driving was relegated to the subconscious mind as it became easy and automatic. You no longer needed to think about the manoeuvres because you did them on autopilot. You were driving subconsciously.

★ ★ ★

When the conscious mind and subconscious mind are in harmony, you truly have willpower. You are 'single-minded'. Using our *Mind Over Fatter* Hypnotherapy download (see page 68), I'm going to help you use your new understanding of how your mind works to change those habits, reverse that negative thinking and end your bad eating patterns forever.

★ ★ ★

'YOUR CONSCIOUS MIND HAS A WILL. BUT IT'S THE SUBCONSCIOUS MIND THAT HAS THE POWER.'

THE POWER OF HYPNOSIS

Mention hypnosis in a conversation and some people will be immediately suspicious. They worry that the hypnotherapist will 'mess with their mind'; that they'll fall too deeply into 'trance' and never come out; or that they'll end up doing something against their will. Other people will proudly announce, 'You'll never be able to hypnotize *me*. I'm not remotely suggestible. Good luck.'

The fact is, 'trance' is something we all experience every single day. When you're engrossed in a film or activity and lose track of time, you are experiencing a state similar to hypnosis. When you drive your car along a familiar route and don't even notice you did it, you are in a state of hypnosis. Trance is a perfectly normal state of mind.

So how exactly does it work? Hypnosis alters our awareness in such a way that our conscious mind is switched off, and our subconscious is made more alert. You are not asleep, and you are not unaware of what's going on around you. In fact, you're in a heightened state of awareness but, because you're relaxed, you're more open to suggestion. It's a kind of sleep of the nervous system where your body is relaxed and your mind receptive. The conscious part of your mind – the logical part – shuts down while the subconscious mind – which is highly suggestive – takes over. Remember I said the subconscious controls 90 per cent of our actions? It is *always* listening.

The subconscious mind is a deep-seated, instinctive force. During hypnosis it listens to the words the therapist is using and uses them to reprogramme negative patterns of behaviour. For example, if I used hypnosis to suggest to someone with a fear of public speaking that they actually enjoy public speaking and are very good at it, then their subconscious mind would accept it and act on this suggestion. But if you gave the same suggestion to them consciously, they would disregard it. That's why we can go blue in the face giving the same advice over and over again to a pal with a problem. You have to get to their subconscious reasoning if you want to change anything.

The word hypnosis originates from Hypnos – the Greek god of sleep. Hypnosis is mentioned in the Bible and was also used in Ancient Egypt to cure women of infertility. But it was not until the 1950s that medical hypnosis began to gain credibility, as research into its many benefits gained validity. More reliable measures of 'hypnotizability' were developed, and Stanford University was the first to establish an accepted yardstick called the Stanford Hypnotic Susceptibility Scales. The Stanford Scales showed that almost everyone can be hypnotized.

Hypnosis works: fact. It can be so effective that it's being used as an important part of healing in some leading hospitals. We know that hypnotherapy has a genuine effect on the functioning of the mind, as well as the body. It is a painless, fast way to change behaviour and has been scientifically proven over and over again.

Our subconscious mind is a wonderful, powerful force. Without us even being aware, it controls the majority of our actions. And the beauty of it is, by changing our mind, we can change our behaviour too.

THE MIND OVER FATTER HYPNOTHERAPY DOWNLOAD

In our free *Mind Over Fatter* download, we're going to use hypnosis to change how you behave around food. The purpose of your hypnotherapy recording is to re-programme the negative eating patterns of both thought and action that originate in your mind and in your belief system. As these negative behaviours are challenged and overcome, you'll find that you become free of the need to overeat, binge and use food as a cure for difficult emotions.

Every single time you play your download you will be reinforcing the message in your subconscious and replacing old, negative suggestions with new powerful, positive ones. As you play the download, the image of you at your ideal weight will become more real and more attainable each time you hear it. When your subconscious mind is able to see the ideal you and to accept you looking that way, then it works hard to make that a reality for you.

As you let go of conscious control of the mind, your subconscious mind takes over. The critical factor shuts down and the mind is able to accept ideas it may have previously rejected. Because your unwanted eating habits have their origins in your subconscious, this is the part that has to change in order for your whole relationship with food to change. Every time you play your download you are reprogramming your subconscious so that old habits are removed and replaced. The analytical part of your mind tunes out and the creative side tunes in.

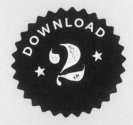

★ ★ ★

HOW WILL IT WORK?

★ ★ ★

★ Go to www.mindoverfatterdownload.co.uk and follow the instructions for the Hypnotherapy download.

★ Find a time when you are on your own, and quiet, just before bed is perfect. *Play the download every day without a break for 14 days*. This is crucial, because the mind learns by repetition. 14 days is enough time for the subconscious to accept the message, seed the new ideas and then begin to make subtle changes in your behaviour.

★ Once the two weeks is up, continue to play the download regularly (at least once a week) to consolidate the message in your subconscious mind.

★ During the hypnosis you will be in an enhanced state of awareness – hearing my voice but not needing to concentrate on it. You will feel relaxed, your breathing will become slower and deeper and your pulse rate will drop. You'll become less interested in events going on around you.

We all change a little differently. Some people notice changes immediately, others notice them bit by bit, or only notice how much they've altered when they look back at how they were before. Just be aware that no matter how significant or small the changes are, *it's all proof that the hypnosis is working.* The differences can be subtle, but powerful. You may notice that you're feeling full more quickly; that you're leaving food on your plate; eating more slowly; or making healthier choices. Your subconscious mind is doing its job beautifully and will carry on working until you reach your ideal weight.

★ ★ ★

HYPNOTHERAPY DOWNLOAD

69

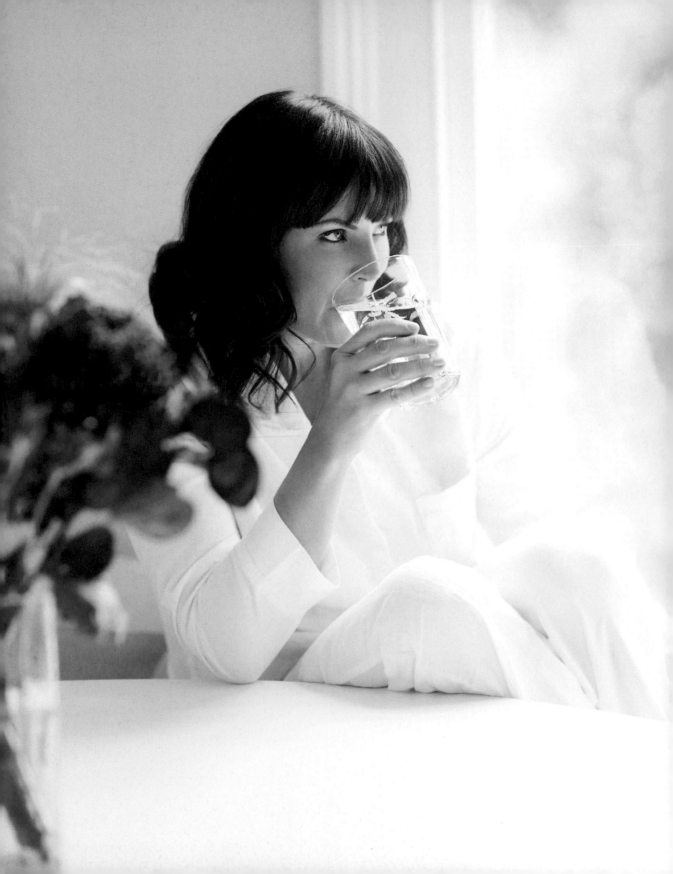

THINK
YOURSELF SLIM

THE SEVEN SECRETS OF SLIM

In Step One: See Yourself Slim, I took you deep into the corners of your subconscious mind. In Step Two: Think Yourself Slim, it's time to recruit your *conscious* mind onto our team. Why? Because your conscious mind is responsible for making 200 food-related decisions every single day.

YOUR CONSCIOUS MIND:

Is your thinking mind

Has no memory

Can only hold one thought at a time

Has four essential functions: it identifiies, compares, analyses and decides

★ ★ ★

It first *identifies* incoming information from your five senses: sound, smell, sight, taste and touch. Imagine waiting to be served in a café. A batch of freshly baked scones is brought out from the kitchen. The smell wafts up your nose; you can see how soft and delicious they look; you can practically taste them.

Next your conscious mind *compares* them with your previous experiences of eating scones. Did you like them? It also compares the experience of eating scones with the experience of eating the other food on offer in the café. Will the scones be more satisfying than the other options?

The brain then *analyses* the information before it *decides*. Your conscious mind can only process 'yes' or 'no'. So as you stare at those scones it does its analysis and has to make a simple decision. Will I have a scone? Yes... or no?

But what you are about to discover is that during this entire process your conscious thinking is secretly being influenced. During each of these cognitive functions your mind is being misinformed, misled and confused by environmental factors.

Forget willpower. Step Two isn't about learning to 'stick with the plan'– it's about becoming savvy about what really drives our decisions around eating. One of my favourite things we filmed for the TV series *Secret Eaters* were the 'secret science' segments. If you watched the show you'll know this is the part where a secret experiment was conducted on members of the public to find out what really makes us eat more. I gained some amazing insights into what drives us – and fools us – when it comes to our eating behaviours. I realized overeating was not about willpower, discipline or self-delusion. We're actually being tricked.

It got me thinking. What if we could use this information and flip it on its head? If there were outside influences making us eat more, what if we were able to bring these to our conscious awareness and use them to our advantage? What if we could trick ourselves into eating less? It would give us the perfect diet. One that we didn't even realise we were following.

It was on the final series of *Secret Eaters* that I first met Dr Christy Fergusson, a psychologist and nutritional therapist. Together we've created the Seven Secrets of Slim. These aren't gimmicks or quick fixes; they're scientifically proven ways to tip the odds in your favour when it comes to losing weight. I want to share these with you because I believe that if you take our advice, you can quite literally *think* yourself slim.

★ 1 ★

PRE-PLAN AND PRE-ORDER

Despite our best intentions to keep our cupboards stocked with healthy food, plan our meals in advance and pack a sensible lunch for work, most of us still make food decisions on the fly. We grab breakfast while rushing to a meeting; decide what to eat for dinner based on what's left in the fridge; and whenever we run out of supplies nip to the shops in a mad dash. If this sounds horribly familiar, then your waistline could be paying the price. Research reveals that when we leave food decisions until we are hungry, we're simply creating a recipe for disaster.

I know, we've all heard it before: 'Don't shop when you're hungry'. But really, *do not shop when you're hungry*. Hunger messes with our ability to make healthy decisions when choosing food. And it's not just you — research has proven that not only do we buy *more* food when our stomach is empty, but we also stock up on *more unhealthy* calorie-laden treats. Hunger influences *all* our decisions around food choices, and there's plenty of evidence to show us how and why.

THE HUNGER MONSTER

In one study, 68 participants were asked to avoid eating for five hours, then go shopping for food. During the study, the food on offer was divided into high-calorie items (such as sweets, crisps, red meat) and low-calorie items (such as fruit, vegetables, chicken breasts). When the time came to go shopping, half the group was offered a plate of crackers to eat until they no longer felt hungry. The study found that those who hadn't eaten for five hours loaded up on more high-calorie foods than those who had been allowed to eat the crackers.

But here is where it gets really interesting: the participants weren't even in a supermarket, they were shopping online. And as more and more of us move into to having groceries delivered, we think we're safe from being tempted by tasty treats on the supermarket shelves. Not so. This study proves that even if you're buying online, hunger will still get the better of you.

DON'T GRAB ON THE GO

Scientific research has shown that if you pre-order your meals, then you can trick yourself into making healthier choices. To put this to the test, the *Secret Eaters* team invited two groups of office workers to take part in a team-building activity and then eat lunch together. Both groups were offered the same selection of foods and could order as much or as little food as they wanted. *But*, one group had to order their lunch straight after breakfast, while the others had to choose what to eat at lunchtime, when they were hungry.

As part of the experiment their leftover food was weighed to calculate which group had eaten the most. As predicted, those who had pre-ordered their meals not only chose healthier options but they also consumed less food. In fact the group that pre-ordered their lunch ate 700 fewer calories overall – a staggering 68 per cent less than those who ate on impulse.

So if you've been grabbing breakfast on the way to work and scoffing it at your desk; if you've been choosing your lunch while waiting in line at the local café; or if you've been deciding what to have for dinner while rummaging around your fridge, then your waistline could be suffering. Don't trust your stomach to make food decisions for you; it's time to let your head take the lead.

★ ★ ★

TOP TIPS

★ Always eat before doing your weekly shop, and follow a pre-written list. Whether you're wandering the aisles in person or shopping online, your hunger will make you more likely to load up on unhealthy treats.

★ Stop making food decisions on the fly. As much as possible, plan your weekly meals when you can think clearly and are not being influenced by an underfed appetite.

★ Pre-order your lunch or take a packed lunch to work so you'll be less tempted by sights and aromas when lunchtime rolls around. Plan your dinner in advance so you aren't making a decision about what to eat when you're already hungry.

★ If you eat out regularly, plan ahead. Most restaurant menus are available to view online. Choose a time when you aren't hungry to check out the options and decide what you are going to have.

✦ ✦ *2* ✦ ✦

MAKE A MEAL OF IT

There was a time when the dining table was the heart of the family. Every evening, children and parents would sit around the kitchen table, share a home-cooked meal together and talk about their day. I can certainly remember being a kid in the 1970s and 1980s when 'tea time' around the table was sacrosanct.

So be honest. How often do you use your dining table now? Has it become a dumping ground for the ironing and bills? Do you prefer to sit in front of the TV with your dinner on your lap?

Flexi-time, shift work, overtime; it's safe to say our working lives are no longer restricted to the familiar 'nine to five' working week. Families now run on different schedules. We eat breakfast alone while our partner sleeps off the night shift; we eat dinner alone while our kids are socializing and our other half is working late. Many of us are single or divorced. It seems that eating on our lonesome has become commonplace, so we don't even bother to buy a dining table anymore.

DEATH OF THE DINNER TABLE

So, as we move away from meals around the table to meals on our lap in front of the TV, the question is: are we eating more? Has the death of the dinner table played a role in our widening waistlines? The theory is that if you sit and eat your meal at the dinner table you count it. Your brain takes note, and considers it a proper meal. As a result you feel fuller and will snack less later.

On *Secret Eaters* I presented an experiment that put this theory to the test. Two families were invited to enjoy a meal together and then play board games afterwards. Crucially, bowls of snacks were placed within easy reach of them to see who would go for them. The first family ate their meal around the table, while the second family sat on the sofa and watched TV as they ate. If the theory was correct, the family who ate in front of the TV would eat more than the family who ate at the dinner table.

At the end of the games, the remaining snack food was weighed to see how much each family had eaten. The results were incredible. The family who ate in front of the TV ate a staggering 98 per cent more food than the family who'd eaten at the dinner table. Could this explain why so many of us overindulge in snacks even when we've just finished a meal?

ACTION-PACKED DISASTER

The death of the dinner table is only part

of the problem. Research also tells us that when you eat in front of the TV, you can also end up eating more depending on the *type* of show you're watching. Yes, you read that correctly. Certain types of shows may actually make you eat more food.

In another study, researchers from the Cornell Food and Brand Lab gave 94 undergraduates chocolate, biscuits, carrots and grapes to eat while watching 20 minutes of TV. A third of the participants watched part of an action movie, a third watched a generic chat show, and the final third watched the same segment from the action movie but on mute.

They found that those undergraduates who watched the action movie ate *twice as much* overall. They took in 98 per cent more food than those watching the chat show. And even those watching the action movie on mute ate 36 per cent more.

Their study shows that the more distracting the programme is in terms of noise, flashing lights, camera cuts and so on, the more we eat. It's obvious when you think about it. When we watch TV, we're distracted, and so we're paying less attention to what and how much we are eating. The more engaging and enthralling the show, the more treacherous it will be for your waistline.

The results speak for themselves, so if you've ditched the dinner table in favour of TV dinners then your waistline will be paying the price. It's time to hit the pause button and get back around the table for meal times.

★ ★ ★

TOP TIPS

★ Even if you're eating alone, sit at the table, turn off your TV and laptop, mute your phone and focus on your meal. Give your body a chance to recognize that you're actually eating something.

★ If you do have to eat in front of the TV, always pre-plate and pre-portion your food beforehand.

★ If you love action-packed movies, crime thrillers and big blockbusters then bring out healthy snacks like nuts and fruit and use the distraction to your advantage.

SIZE MATTERS

What if I told you that overeating has little to do with feeling hungry and is more to do with your environment – would you believe me?

In fact, there is an increasing body of evidence that proves that environmental factors are more likely to make you eat and drink greater quantities than real physiological hunger. I'm not talking about how sunny it is, or whether it's raining (again) – but immediate environmental cues in your surroundings. Things like how tall your drinking glass is, how big the packet is that you are holding, how deep your spoon is and wait for it… how big or small your dinner plate is. These *all* have an impact on how much you're going to consume.

It's a real irony that in the 21st century we resort to radical surgery to curb our overeating and spend a fortune on diet books trying to work out why we're overweight – when all along there's a culprit lurking in our kitchen cupboard in the form of an oversized dinner plate.

It may seem a little hard to swallow… so don't just take my word for it, let's look at the facts. In the 1950s, the average dinner plate was 23 centimetres in diameter. Then slowly over the decades, it began to grow. By the 1980s it had increased to 28 centimetres, and now it's a supersize whopper at 33 centimetres. That's about a 45 per cent increase in size. It's no surprise then that as our dinner plates have grown, so have we. In fact, the increase in the rate of obesity we've seen over the last 60 years is in direct parallel with the increase in the size of our dinner plate. Coincidence? I don't think so.

DO YOU LIKE A BIG PACKAGE?

Bigger is better, right? Wrong. Here's the problem with a big package – and it may seem blindingly obvious – bigger packets of food make us eat more.

When food is wrapped in small packets, we slow down our compulsive eating simply because it makes us consciously think about what we're doing. Bigger packets of food may save us money and endless trips to the supermarket, but ultimately they lead to larger meals. And what happens when we're faced with a larger meal? We eat it.

In one experiment, 40 adults were invited to watch a video at a parent-teacher meeting. Each of the viewers was given a bag of M&M's to munch on. Some were handed a 230-gram bag, the rest a 460-gram bag. Afterwards, the researcher weighed how much was left in the bags. The results were striking. Those who were given the bigger bag ate, on average, 71 more M&M's than those who had the bag that was half the size. That's *twice* as many – and more importantly, a significant 264 extra calories.

If I gave you a big packet of spaghetti you'd cook more; if I gave you a big jar of sauce you'd pour more; and if I gave you a big packet of biscuits you'd most likely eat them all. It's the same with drinking glasses. If I handed you a tall, skinny glass and a short, wide glass, you would drink 25–30 per cent more from the wide one.

The reason we do this is because we use the size of the packet as a reference to work out what we think a 'normal' amount to eat is. And food manufacturers use this to their advantage by manipulating us to eat more of their product. They set a new 'normal' amount to eat by making their packaging bigger.

Use a bigger packet, box, jar, plate or glass and you could eat 20 per cent more. Use a smaller packet, box, jar, plate or glass and you could eat 20 per cent less. If you want to stop overeating, you need to tip the odds in your favour. Size does matter. And what you do with it counts.

★ ★ ★

TOP TIPS

★ Downsize bowls, plates and dishes. You eat with your eyes, not your stomach. So if you want to reduce your portion size and still feel satisfied you need to use smaller plates and bowls. The smaller the serving dish, the less you will eat.

★ Trick yourself slim: make this work for you by serving salads on large plates and more calorie-laden foods on small plates.

★ Opt for tall, slim glasses over wider ones if you have a calorific drink, but go for the wide glasses if you want to increase your daily water intake.

★ Resist buying family-sized packets, jars, boxes and tins of food. The bigger it is, the more likely it is you'll eat more.

★★★★ 4 ★★★★

OUT OF SIGHT OUT OF MIND . . . AND IN SIGHT IN MIND

How many times have you started the week with great intentions, only to have your resolve collapse in the face of temptation? It all begins so well doesn't it? You order a big grocery shop, stock your cupboards with healthy food and even plan your meals for the week. You are set for success.

But then you go into work only to discover that your colleague has spent the weekend baking (even though she's on a diet) and has perched a box of cakes by the photocopier for the whole office to share…

You are now officially caught in the 'see food' trap. If you see it, you want it, and psychology dictates that it won't be long before your willpower waivers and next thing you know, you've eaten three muffins. Oops.

WHY YOU CAN'T RESIST

If you've been beating yourself up about not having enough willpower or not being disciplined enough, then *stop*. It just so happens that willpower has nothing to do with it – you're actually physiologically designed to start feeling hungry simply by *thinking* about food.

Most of us have heard of Pavlov's dogs, which were conditioned to salivate at the mere ringing of a bell. Why? Because it triggered the anticipation of food. When we hear, see or smell something we consider tasty, our body kicks into action. That's why when you watch any of the countless TV shows about food, buffered by advertisements selling food, your mouth starts to water.

Just the thought of something delicious is enough to make your pancreas begin to secrete insulin. This chemical helps the body metabolize the impending sugar rush your brain has in mind. What it also does is make you feel hungry by lowering your blood sugar levels. So simply thinking about food is enough to make you feel hungry for it.

IS IT CALLING YOUR NAME?

To prove this theory, psychologists carried out a fascinating study using a group of secretaries, an office and a jar of chocolates. Each week, the clear sweet jar was moved to a different spot.

During the first week, a secretary would find the sweet jar at the corner of her desk. The next week, it was in her top left-hand drawer. And on the last week, it was on her filing cabinet a couple of metres from her desk.

You can guess what happened. When the

sweet jar was placed on the desk (where the secretary had to look at it all day) she ate more chocolates. In fact, on average, each secretary ate nine chocolates when they were right in front of her. That's around 225 calories. If she had to go to the hassle of opening the desk drawer she ate around six chocolates, and if she had to get up and walk to get a chocolate then she only ate four.

The more hassle it is to eat something, the less likely we are to eat it. If we had to press a lever a hundred times for a mini-cupcake, then we wouldn't eat as many. If you had to climb to the top of a flight of stairs for a biscuit then you'd soon work out it's not worth the effort.

But is it just about convenience? It turns out that when the researchers quizzed the secretaries afterwards, they told them that when they had two metres between them and the chocolate it gave them enough time to talk themselves out of having any more. Whereas when the chocolate was in reaching distance, the interval between impulse and reason was too short.

Now that you know about the effect of food proximity on your appetite, start thinking about how to make it work in your favour. Many of us downplay its importance, but research proves that you'll consume more calories if unhealthy food is convenient.

So next time your work colleague brings treats into the office, ask them to put them out of sight. That way, they're out of mind too.

★ ★ ★
TOP TIPS

★ Is your fresh fruit stuffed at the bottom of your fridge in the 'rotting drawer'? Get it out and display it in a fruit bowl where you can easily see it and eat it.

★ Don't keep sweets, chocolate, biscuits and ice cream in the house. If the craving hits, you're less likely to leave the house and buy it. Stock your kitchen with healthy treats instead, so that it's easier to grab something nutritious.

★ Take healthy snacks to work and keep them close at hand.

THE 20-MINUTE RULE

It sounds simple enough: eat until you're satisfied… and then stop. If we just tuned into our bodies and finished when we'd had enough, we wouldn't overeat surely? Obvious in theory. But it turns out that our bodies may actually be tricking us into eating more than we really need.

Most of us eat until we feel full, and that signal tells us we've consumed enough. But what if there was a way you could create this feeling of fullness by eating less? It means we could cut calories and still feel satisfied as opposed to deprived. It may sound too good to be true but science proves it. Welcome to the facts behind the '20-minute rule'.

MEALTIME MONSTER

Let's consider a typical mealtime. We sit down, fork in hand, our eyes on the prize, and then the mindless eating begins. Be honest, do you practically inhale your meals, chow down your food and then load up on second helpings before the first bite even hits your stomach? If you eat fast, you're not alone. Many of us eat like we're never going to encounter food again. We scoff down our meals at lightning speed and then our brains are left doing a double-take trying to work out what just happened.

You may not have given it much thought before, but it takes approximately 20 minutes for your brain to register that your stomach is full. So if your meals become a memory within seconds and you're helping yourself to more before your body knows what's hit it, then you *will* overeat. We're simply not giving our bodies the chance to go through their natural signalling process.

MEET YOUR MESSENGERS

To understand this process a little better, we need to understand our biochemistry. That feeling of 'fullness' we have is entirely dependent on a variety of chemical feedback loops between our gut and our brain.

Our hormones are our 'satiety messengers', telling our brain that enough is enough. The problem? Most of us are racing through our meals so fast that our stomach is beating those fullness messengers to the finish line and we're left with that uncomfortable 'stuffed' feeling.

So how does this vicious cycle start? The 'hunger hormone' ghrelin is produced mostly by the stomach and acts directly on the brain's pleasure centres. But if we want to eat less and still feel satisfied we need to utilize the hormone leptin. Leptin is the arch enemy of ghrelin and works by directly suppressing hunger, stopping us overeating.

SALSA AND SECOND HELPINGS

I saw this theory proven on *Secret Eaters*. The producers invited a group of unsuspecting participants along to a salsa club for a dance class and then some lunchtime tapas.

Of course they weren't really interested in their dancing skills, what they actually wanted to know was this: would the group given a 20-minute break between the first and second helpings of tapas eat less and consume fewer calories than the group who were allowed to eat continuously? Both groups were given the same menu. The first group was continuously offered more food throughout their meal. The second, on the other hand, had to wait 20 minutes before being offered seconds.

After everyone had finished eating we weighed up the leftover food and calculated which group had eaten the most. As predicted, those who constantly helped themselves to seconds ate more than those who had to wait 20 minutes before having another helping. In fact, the group that waited ate 10 per cent less than their peers.

The science proves it. Slowing down and waiting is the secret to eating less and still feeling satisfied.

★ ★ ★

TOP TIPS

★ Practise mindful eating. Take time to think about what you are eating: the colours, the aromas and the taste. Take your time.

★ If you think you want second helpings wait until your meal has started to digest and your brain has had time to catch up.

★ Chew your food. The chewing process is vital for adequate digestion and healthy portion control.

★ Avoid mindlessly shovelling in food. Sit at a table with no distraction and focus on your food.

★ Put small quantities on your fork, and put it down between mouthfuls.

THINK BEFORE YOU DRINK

I have a confession to make. I've discovered a bit of a passion for wine. I've also discovered a bit of a passion for vodka. And gin. And I won't say no to a cocktail if you're offering. The problem is, when I've had the wine, gin, vodka and cocktail I then fall face first into a doner kebab. And I know I'm not alone, people! That's right, who hasn't eaten yesterday's curry when they've got a killer hangover?

Here's the thing: we know a moderate amount of alcohol can actually increase longevity, so it can't all be doom and gloom, but do we really need to avoid alcohol if we're serious about losing weight? Does booze *really* make us eat more food? The fact is that yes, it does. And it's not just about lowered inhibitions – according to scientists, alcohol actually has a physiological effect on our appetite.

BEER BRAIN

So how does this happen? When we drink, our body doesn't store alcohol in the same way that it does food. Remember, alcohol is a toxin, so to keep it from having too much of a toxic impact on our system the body has to metabolize the alcohol as an energy source. In order to facilitate that process our glycogen (carbohydrate) stores become depleted. Cue the carbohydrate cravings. And hello chips!

Alcohol is also a diuretic. Not only does it have us constantly running to the toilet, but it also decreases our levels of electrolytes, such as sodium. As our sodium levels drop, the salt cravings kick in – and before we know it we're loading the chips with salt, cheese and ketchup. Your mind isn't playing tricks on you. That white bread really does taste better with that glass of wine.

'AND IT'S NOT JUST ABOUT
LOWERED INHIBITIONS –
ACCORDING TO SCIENTISTS, ALCOHOL
ACTUALLY HAS A PHYSIOLOGICAL
EFFECT ON OUR APPETITE. '

We eat more because alcohol affects our appetite. Full stop. It messes with our blood sugar levels, depletes our energy stores and even switches off the satiety hormone that tells our brain when to stop. So it's not really surprising we find ourselves ordering a Big Mac after a few glasses of wine.

But it can't all be physiological can it? Lowered inhibitions must surely play a role? If we make a couple of hundred food-related decisions every day, it's inevitable our judgement about what to eat, and how much, will be influenced when we're under the influence.

While chomping chips at 4 a.m. might not be the best idea, there's another health issue at work. Your weight. Drinking messes with your appetite, kicks your cravings into overdrive and can have your brain making important decisions about food with its beer goggles on. If you're trying to whittle that waistline then please remember – think before you drink.

★ ★ ★

TOP TIPS

★ If you're heading out for the evening nominate yourself as the designated driver. Even when you're tempted you'll have to stay strong and abstain.

★ Shift your mindset. Don't make a song and dance about reducing your alcohol consumption. See avoiding alcohol as a positive step towards reaching your weight-loss goal.

★ Now you know that alcohol messes with your appetite, be aware that if you're tempted by a tipple it'll probably cause you to eat more. Is it worth ditching the diet for?

★ Trick your taste buds by smearing gin or vodka around the top of your glass before filling it with a low-calorie mixer. That way, you can 'smell' the alcohol and trick yourself into thinking you're having the real deal.

TIRED AND HUNGRY

We've all heard the weight-loss mantra 'exercise more, eat less'. But there's another, more overlooked, formula we should also be paying attention to – '*sleep* more, eat less'.

Sleep plays a crucial role in regulating our body, but sadly our generation aren't very good at bagging the right amount of zeds. In fact, we sleep around 20–25 per cent less than our grandparents did at our age. Since sleep debt is cumulative, this amounts to more than a full night's sleep lost every single week.

We all know that a lack of sleep makes us cranky and unfocused, but less understood is the effect it has on our waistlines. One of the features I presented for *Secret Eaters* was an undercover sleep experiment. Eight volunteers took part in what *they* thought was a study investigating the link between sleep deprivation and mental performance. Unbeknownst to them, what was *actually* being studied was the link between a poor night's sleep and poor food choices.

Four of the subjects were allowed to get a decent night's sleep; the other four were woken up at 1 a.m., then 4 a.m. and asked to take an IQ test.

The next morning, all eight volunteers were given snack bags with the same snack options inside. At the end of the day what had been eaten was analysed. The results were shocking. The sleep-deprived group ate a whopping 35 per cent more calories than those who had been left undisturbed during the night. Proof that a lack of sleep leads to munching on higher calorie and higher fat options the following day.

DAZED AND CONFUSED

When you're tired, your impulse control and judgement is affected – your brain doesn't want to conjure up exciting recipes or analyse the healthiest option. That's why we reach for the nearest snack, or find it harder to resist when offered that high-calorie treat at breakfast time. Our brain is a computer, and when it's run down, it makes skewed choices. Obvious, when you think about it.

SLEEP YOURSELF SLIM

Missing precious hours of sleep doesn't just affect mental clarity, it also directly affects your body, messing with your metabolism and slowing your ability to burn fuel. It disrupts the essential hormones that regulate blood sugar levels and process fat. So tiredness not only leads us to make poorer nutritional choices, it also makes our bodies less equipped to deal with the effects of those high-calorie foods we choose. It's a fact that when we sleep well, we tend to snack less.

But improving your sleep to improve your waistline isn't simply about getting more hours in bed. It's also about the *quality* of rest – making sure you have proper, undisturbed sleep.

★ ★ ★

TOP TIPS

★ If your mind is busy and active at night, try meditation. There are plenty of courses and downloads. Meditation has been proven to be effective for relaxation.

★ Aim to get at least 30 minutes of sunlight every day. This will increase your vitamin D levels, which can help improve sleep.

★ Avoid watching TV or sitting at a computer for at least one hour before bedtime.

★ Exercise during the day for between 30 and 60 minutes as this can help improve sleep. However, be wary of exercising too late at night, as this can delay the release of melatonin, preventing you from falling asleep.

★ Opt for lighter meals in the evening.

★ Create a healthy sleeping environment. Keep your bedroom quiet, dark and cool.

★ If you do struggle to drift off, don't lie tossing and turning for more than 30 minutes. Get up, read a book and relax elsewhere until you feel sleepy. This way, you don't associate your bed with a place you can't sleep.

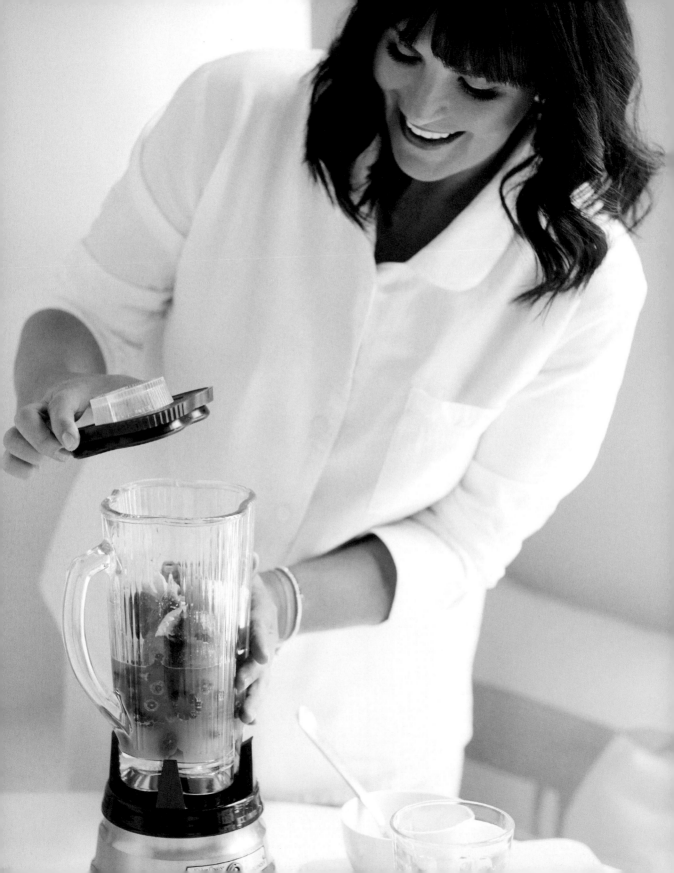

STEP

3

★★★ ★★★

EAT
YOURSELF SLIM

FEEDING YOUR BODY

As I mentioned at the very start of our journey, the best and most effective way to use this book is as a three-step process.

In Step One: See Yourself Slim we explored the power of your unconscious mind and how to utilize it to get the strong, healthy body you were born to have. By listening to your hypnotherapy download every day, you are already making powerful subconscious changes to how you eat.

In Step Two: Think Yourself Slim, we discovered how our conscious minds get tricked into overeating. By taking on board our tips in the Seven Secrets of Slim you'll be able to use what science has revealed about psychology to help you 'think' your way into being a better, slimmer you.

These first two steps were designed to change what you feed your mind. In Step Three: Eat Yourself Slim, we're going to focus on what you feed your body. It's the final cherry on the cake. Even though you're not meant to be eating cake...

What you feed your body is absolutely key to your long-term health and well-being. There's so much more to life than obsessing about food – but if you don't properly nourish your body and be mindful about what you eat, it can have a domino effect on all aspects of your life. Ever had that massive plate of cheesy pasta at lunch and then felt sleepy around 3 p.m.? Yup. Felt sick after too many bags of cheese and onion crisps? I have. Or not wanted to undress in front of your partner because your belly's bigger than your boobs? Been there, bought the control pants. As you begin to take back control of your eating (perhaps for the first time in your life) you'll find yourself naturally drawn

to the right foods to fuel that wonderful, complex machine –
your body. You'll start to eat to live – *not* live to eat.

So what can you expect? I've worked with a team of expert
home economists to create 60 gorgeous, healthy and nutritious
recipes for you to pick and choose from. This isn't an elimination
diet, instead each recipe is gently calorie controlled, but more
importantly balanced and nutritious, to encourage optimum
health and weight.

If you're the kind of person who appreciates structure then
I've provided a simple 14-day healthy-eating plan for you, using
the recipes provided. If you're the kind of person who prefers
to freestyle, then great – just make your own choices from each
section. And if you're the kind of person who just loves a recipe
book full of inspirational food, then be my guest – these meals
are designed to be enjoyed by the whole family too. All I ask is
that you enjoy three square meals a day: breakfast, lunch and
dinner. And, if you need a snack to keep your blood sugar levels
even and your moods and energy steady, we've given you plenty
of easy ideas to try as well as some great recipes.

Step Three is your final power tool for change. This isn't
some faddy weight-loss diet; it's common-sense, back-to-basics,
wholesome eating. In other words, an investment in your health
and happiness. Enjoy it.

FOOD ON THE BRAIN

It's true, I have a library of diet books on my kitchen shelf. And I know only too well how 'healthy-eating plans' can sometimes seem like a punishment. I mean, who really wants to give up their nightly chocolate treat in front of the TV, or that soothing bottle of wine after a tough day at work? I get it... food is our comfort. But we also owe it to ourselves to be educated about what we're putting into our body – after all, it's the only one we've got.

The team on Mind Over Fatter have worked really hard to create healthy, wholesome meals that will nourish you. We've also worked hard not to make this a tough 'elimination' diet. We've included a little dairy, some natural sugar, and believe in using oils. Stuff most of us eat every day anyway. Or should.

I'm a big believer in 'everything in moderation', but who are we kidding, we're all creatures of habit living on the same foods day in, day out. Just think about your breakfast. Tell the truth. The chances are you have the same thing most days. Toast, cereal, milk, tea, coffee, sugar – or a variation of.

Our modern diet has a few key culprits: sugar, wheat, dairy, alcohol and caffeine. We may fool ourselves into believing we have a varied diet, but when it comes down to it most of us are just eating too much of the list above.

So I wanted to include a brief chapter on how these main players can really mess with you physiologically. That way, you can decide for yourself how far you want to go in cleaning up your diet – and whether you'd prefer to avoid some things altogether in the future.

The choice is yours.

SUGAR

For years we've been obsessed by the low-fat mantra and the mistaken belief that 'fat makes us fat'. We're so busy scouring food packets for the low-fat label that we've forgotten one crucial ingredient: sugar. Our body converts sugar into fat. I could hand you a bin bag full of sugar and slap a '100 per cent fat free' label on the side; it would be accurate and you might think this meant it would have little effect on your weight. The reality, however, is that sugar converts to glucose in our bodies. And what happens to excess glucose when we don't burn it off? We store it as *fat*.

So, when you're looking at food packaging make sure you look out for words like aspartame, sucralose, dextrose, malt, sucrose, corn syrup and glucose. They're all sugars. And remember sugar by any other name is still as sweet. Be realistic, and think about reducing your intake.

WHEAT

I know, it tastes amazing right? That warm hunk of crusty white bread, dipped in olive oil. The problem is that wheat contains gluten, a protein that can wreak havoc on your digestive system. If you find yourself bloating up after meals, then gluten could be the culprit. If you want to whittle your waist, then try cutting out wheat.

CAFFEINE

It's 7 a.m.. Is the only thought keeping you from hitting the snooze button that double espresso? If you want to curb those crazy food cravings you need to balance your natural energy, stabilize your blood sugar levels and soothe your stress. When you throw caffeine into the mix this can become an impossible challenge. Ever felt 'tired and wired' all at the same time? Take it slow, wean yourself off gently, and move over to healthy caffeine-free options.

DAIRY

We are a nation raised on dairy. Milk, cheese, butter: all part of our childhoods and a daily fact of life. But did you know that after the age of two many of us don't have the enzyme required to digest lactose? When we do eat it, we can end up feeling bloated and tired as our system tries to cope. Dairy is also addictive. It contains chemicals called casomorphins that lock into the opiate receptors in our brain, creating an almost drug-like effect on us. That's why that night-time cup of cocoa feels so damn good.

ALCOHOL

As you know from the Seven Secrets of Slim in Step Two, cutting back on alcohol is vital if you want to control your weight. Anyone who's experienced a hangover knows that alcohol messes with your mind as well as your body. It's a toxin. A toxin that interferes with hormone production and blood sugar levels, leading to food cravings and weight gain. Gram for gram it's second only to pure fat in terms of calories too. That gut isn't called a 'beer belly' for nothing.

It's time to expand your eating repertoire. The more you introduce a larger variety of foods into your diet, get creative and experiment with natural fresh whole foods, the less reliant you'll become on the processed mulch you were hooked on before. And your body… and mind… will thank you for it.

DITCH THE SABOTEURS

Most of us spend an awful lot of time in our kitchen. So it makes sense that if it isn't a 'healthy' kitchen, both in terms of the food you store there and the *way* you store it, then it shouldn't really be a surprise when you end up with unhealthy eating habits. A mindful kitchen is the first step to a mindful menu.

To create a mindful kitchen, start by eliminating foods that are secretly sabotaging you. Set your kitchen up for success by transforming it into a healthy eating sanctuary. To make this simple, here's a 'ditch it' list to help you get started.

★ Refined carbohydrates: it's time to get rid of the white wheat pasta, white bread, pastries, biscuits, chocolates, cakes.

★ Refined sugars and artificial sweeteners: steer clear and/or bin any processed foods that include in the ingredient list any of the sugars I listed earlier, artificial flavourings or colourings.

★ Processed products: throw out bottled and jarred sauces, such as tomato and pasta sauces or curry sauces, and any ready meals.

★ Dairy: avoid anything full-fat, stick to skimmed or semi-skimmed milk, choose low-fat or 0 per cent fat yoghurt when cooking the recipes and avoid having lots of cheese in the fridge.

★ Stimulants: think about removing coffee and caffeinated tea, and all alcohol – wine, beer, spirits – from your cupboards.

A MINDFUL KITCHEN

Once you've cleared out the rubbish, organize your kitchen so that it helps you, rather than hinders you. Here's some ideas based on the ingredients used in our recipes.

★ Nuts and seeds: pumpkin seeds, sunflower seeds, whole almonds, pistachios, ground almonds, chia seeds, pine nuts, flaked almonds, cashew nuts, pecan nuts.

★ Dried fruit: pitted dates, raisins, prunes, figs, sultanas.

★ Pulses: we've used red lentils and Puy lentils, but all types of lentil are great to have in your store cupboard.

★ Wholegrain carbohydrates: rye bread, wholegrain and seeded pitta bread and tortilla, spelt flour, jumbo oats, porridge oats, brown rice, brown basmati rice, soba or buckwheat noodles, spelt pasta, quinoa.

★ Tinned goods: Keep a stash of quality tinned goods to hand: chopped tomatoes, tuna, cannellini beans, Puy lentils, butter beans, organic coconut milk, black beans, pinto beans, kidney beans, tomato passata, haricot beans and chickpeas are great stand-bys and are all used in these recipes.

★ Oils: we've used a variety of oils in our recipes as it helps to add flavour. However, it's important to think about how much you're using – just one tablespoon of olive oil contains a whopping 120 calories. You can cut down by swapping to an olive oil spray, as we've suggested in many of the recipes, which will mean you use less – as long as you don't go mad with the spray! Other tips are to use a non-stick pan to dry-fry with a little water or to wipe the base of the pan round with kitchen paper to mop up any excess. Get into the habit of measuring the oil you use, and remember once heated it warms and liquefies more so you don't need as much as you think.

★ Sugars: upgrade the sugars and sweeteners in your cupboards to more natural alternatives such as agave syrup, honey and maple syrup. Be mindful when using them – a little drizzle will add more than enough flavour if you need to sweeten and balance a savoury sauce.

★ Fruit and vegetables: stock your fridge with fresh fruit, vegetables and leafy greens. Remove all plastic wrapping and wash before putting them in the fridge, so you can quickly grab what you need. Pick a selection for your fruit bowl at the beginning of each day. Stock up on plain frozen vegetables. Frozen berries are good freezer staples too – great for last-minute smoothies. Larger fruit like melon and mango can be chopped and frozen in portion-sized bags so you'll only eat what you need to. These are fab when that need for something sweet hits you later in the evening.

★ Meat and fish: fill your freezer with fish such as salmon, prawns, cod or other firm white fish fillets, and free-range skinless, boneless chicken breasts and mini fillets.

★ Hot drinks: buy herbal teas such as lemon and ginger, camomile, valerian, peppermint, green and redbush tea to swap with your regular brew. Choose decaffeinated coffee to help you switch from that morning pick-me-up.

★ Herbs: keep fresh herbs on your window ledge or if possible plant a couple of varieties outside. You don't need a lot of space – if you don't have a garden, put them in window boxes and water daily. Herbs freeze well too. Finely chop and pack them into ice cube trays so they are ready to add to the recipes.

Stock up on some glass jars. Fill them up with dried staples so all your healthy options are visible.

Preparing food ahead makes it so much easier to choose a healthy option. It's a good idea to freeze and store some pre-prepared homemade meals like soups, stews, casseroles and curries for emergency dinners. On the recipes we've made suggestions for freezing. And make sure you have plenty of sealable plastic boxes for taking lunches and snacks with you to work.

By following these simple strategies you will not only de-convenience unhealthy foods, but you will also make eating healthy, wholesome foods the easy option.

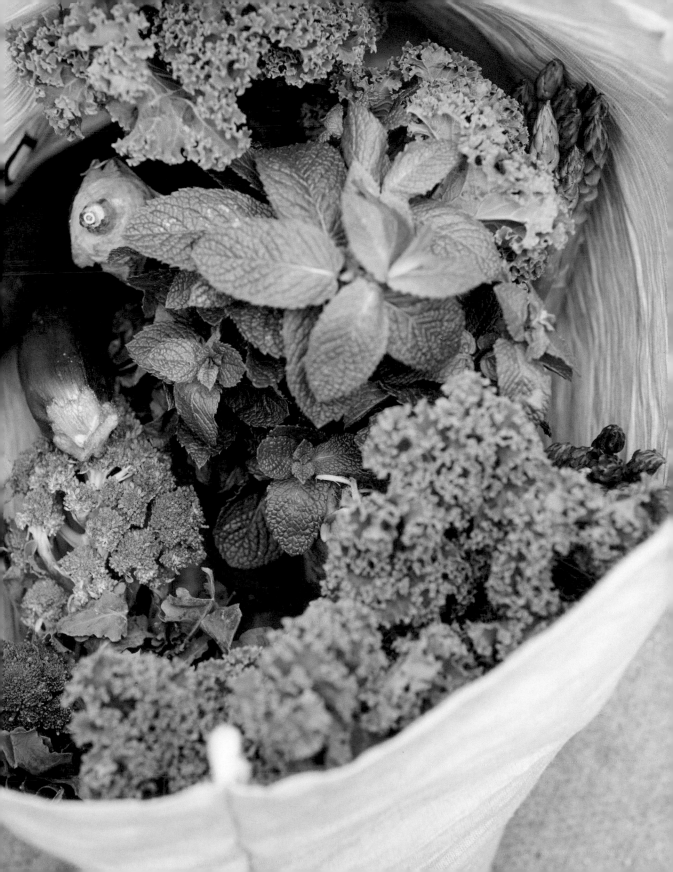

THE MIND OVER FATTER 14-DAY HEALTHY-EATING PLAN

There are lots of recipes in the book for you to cherry-pick from to pull together your own signature diet. If, however, you like to follow rules, we've worked out this healthy-eating plan with suggestions for breakfast, lunch, dinner and a quick snack to make it really easy to follow. There are time-saving tips, too, so you know when and how to prepare certain recipes ahead.

If you're vegetarian, swap the meat or fish with tofu, quorn or other meat alternatives.

WEEK 1

★ ★ ★

MONDAY
Breakfast: Berry and vanilla smoothie
Lunch: Chipotle chicken with quick pickled cabbage (cook the chicken the day before if you need to, then store in the fridge overnight)
Snack: Six whole almonds
Dinner: Veggie pilaf with caramelized onions

TUESDAY
Breakfast: Blueberry and pistachio Bircher
Lunch: Japanese crunchy veg noodles with tofu (make the night before and chill; add the mint just before eating)
Snack: Two oatcakes, each spread with a teaspoon of unsweetened peanut butter
Dinner: Tandoori fish with quick veg thoran

WEDNESDAY
Breakfast: Breakfast sundae
Lunch: Hot green bean and feta salad
(steam the vegetables and toast the pine nuts, then assemble
the salad in the morning before work if you need to)
Snack: One banana
Dinner: Veggie two-bean chilli with apple and red onion salsa

THURSDAY
Breakfast: Simple Green Smoothie
Lunch: Shredded cumin chicken with mango and chilli salad
(cook the chicken the night before then cool and chill)
Snack: Eight walnuts
Dinner: Lentil and sweet potato stew

FRIDAY
Breakfast: Dairy-free date and apple porridge
Lunch: Kale and roasted red veg salad (prepare and roast
vegetables for the salad the night before; prepare the
dressing then stir in just before eating)
Snack: One apple
Dinner: Spanish-style fish pie

SATURDAY
Breakfast: Huevos rancheros
Lunch: Mexican street food tacos with quick coriander salsa
Snack: Small handful of kale crisps
Dinner: My favourite ragu with spelt pasta

SUNDAY
Breakfast: Avocado and bacon on rye toast
Lunch: Spicy harissa prawns with lemon quinoa
Snack: One square of the date bar, plus mint tea if you like
Dinner: Whole roast chicken with hot green salad

WEEK 2

★ ★ ★

MONDAY
Breakfast: No-sugar granola stash (serve with an 80-calorie allowance of yogurt or milk)
Lunch: Smoked chicken and grapefruit cups (prepare the chicken filling the night before, but don't add the avocado. Pack in a box with a little gem, wrap the avocado separately then add to the salad just before eating)
Snack: One banana
Dinner: Hot roast vegetable curry

TUESDAY
Breakfast: Ricotta, banana and honey on rye toast
Lunch: Best-ever roast tomato soup (make the soup over the weekend and keep chilled)
Snack: One apple
Dinner: Honey and wholegrain mustard roast salmon with lemon and dill bashed potatoes

WEDNESDAY
Breakfast: Blueberry and pistachio Bircher
Lunch: Roasted vegetable and Puy lentil salad (roast the vegetables in the oven underneath the salmon the night before)
Snack: One pear
Dinner: Roast cod with herby seed crust and curried parsnip mash

THURSDAY
Breakfast: Breakfast sundae
Lunch: Tuna and white bean salad
Snack: One orange
Dinner: Wasabi salmon and peas with roasted sweet potato

FRIDAY
Breakfast: Scrambled egg and tomato on rye toast
Lunch: Sweet potato soup with toasted seeds (make the soup at the weekend and freeze; toast the seeds and store in an airtight container)
Snack: Small bunch of grapes
Dinner: Lean Asian beef burger with shredded salad or the Ultimate veggie burger

SATURDAY
Breakfast: Smoked salmon and spinach spelt pancakes
Lunch: Hot green bean and feta salad
Snack: One square of fig, orange and pecan flapjack (thawed from the freezer)
Dinner: Steamed yoghurt chicken and cumin rice with spicy tomato salad

SUNDAY
Breakfast: Huevos rancheros
Lunch: Vietnamese summer rolls with spicy peanut dipping sauce
Snack: Small portion of Homemade hummus with vegetable crudités
Dinner: Lamb tagine with potatoes and peas

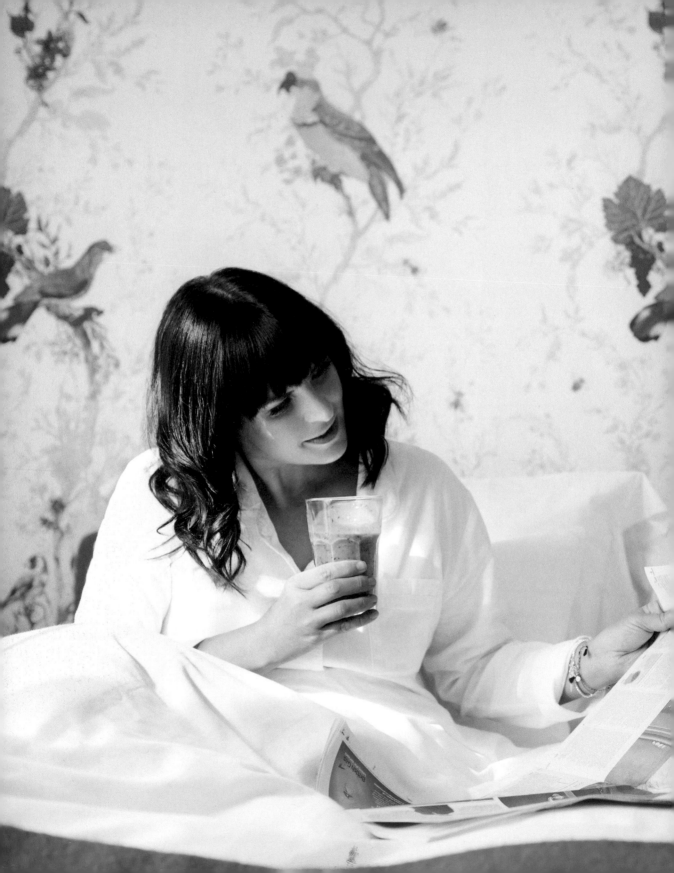

BREAKFASTS

Everyone has an opinion about breakfast. In one camp, there are those who wake up ravenous and like to eat like a king at 7.00 a.m. And in the other, those who can't face a crumb until mid-morning.

I must admit, I used to be one of the latter. The idea of food would make me feel queasy, and I secretly delighted in the mistaken idea that I was somehow saving on calories. But I've learnt, again and again, that having a small meal when you wake up is crucial. It revs up your metabolism, stabilizes your blood sugar, and prevents you needing sugary snacks mid-morning.

So, whether you love it or loathe it, get into it. All of my gorgeous breakfasts are healthy and filling — and still under 300 calories.

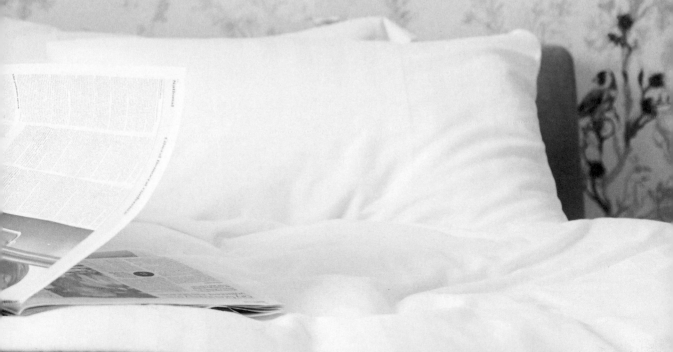

AVOCADO AND BACON
ON RYE TOAST

SERVES

60g (about 2 rashers) smoked back bacon

100g rye bread (2 large slices or 4 small slices, max 190 calories)

1 tablespoon (20g) lemon curd
½ medium avocado, mashed

It's not surprising that avocado on toast has had a surge in popularity recently; not only is it easy to prepare but avocados are packed full of nutrients and good fats which help us feel satisfied after eating. To bring it to a whole new level of luxe, add a scraping of lemon curd and a rasher of bacon – fabulous for a weekend treat.

* * *

You can cook the bacon using your preferred method but here it's microwaved as no extra fat is required and it really intensifies the flavour – plus minimal washing up! If you dry fry or grill it, make sure you blot it on kitchen roll afterwards to absorb any excess fat.

* * *

1 Separate the rashers of bacon and lay them flat on a double thickness of kitchen paper and top with another double thickness of kitchen paper, place this on a microwaveable plate and microwave on the highest setting for 2–3 minutes, checking frequently in the last minute.

2 Meanwhile toast the slices of rye bread in the toaster and spread with the lemon curd.

3 Top each slice with the mashed avocado and, using scissors, snip the bacon bits on top.

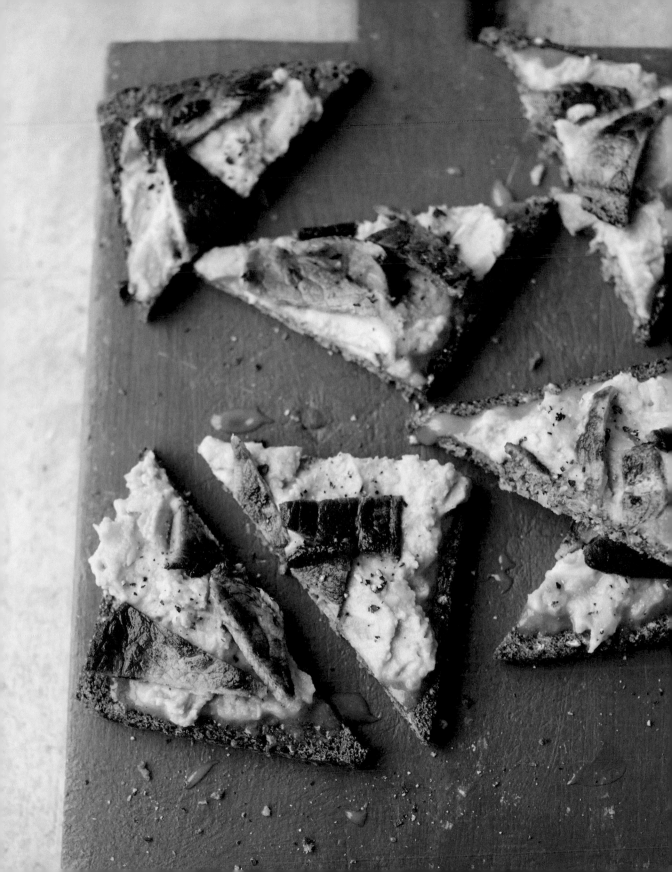

HUEVOS RANCHEROS

SERVES

2

For the sauce
100% mild and light olive
    oil spray
1 medium red onion, sliced
1 large or 2 small red
    peppers, seeds removed,
    thinly sliced
1 clove garlic, thinly sliced

½ teaspoon sweet smoked
    paprika or chipotle
    chilli powder
1 x 400g tin chopped
    tomatoes
pinch of flaked sea salt,
    such as Maldon
freshly ground black pepper

To finish
2 medium free-range eggs
pinch of flaked sea salt,
    such as Maldon
freshly ground black pepper
few sprigs fresh coriander

This gorgeous breakfast is perfect for weekends or a lazy brunch. It also makes a great supper when you can eat the whole thing to yourself!

* * *

You can make a double batch of sauce and keep it in the fridge for two days. Alternatively, let it cool after step 1, divide it into batches and keep the spare in the freezer for up to three months. Thaw overnight in the fridge, then reheat gently, adding a splash of water if the sauce is too thick.

* * *

1 Spray a large non-stick frying pan with olive oil and place over a medium heat. Add the onion, pepper and garlic and fry for 5 minutes until softened. Stir in the smoked paprika and tomatoes. Fill the tomato tin about a quarter full of water to rinse it round and then add to the pan. Simmer for 10–15 minutes until the sauce is rich and thick and any excess water has evaporated. Add salt and pepper to taste.

2 Crack one egg into a cup. Make a small well in the sauce and gently lower the egg into the well. Repeat with the second egg. Season the eggs with a little salt and pepper. Cover the pan with a lid (if you don't have a lid big enough you can use a baking tray). Cook for 3 minutes or until the yolks are just firm.

3 Scatter with coriander and serve.

DAIRY-FREE DATE AND APPLE PORRIDGE

SERVES

2

80g jumbo oats
300ml unsweetened
   soya milk

20g dried dates, chopped
½ teaspoon vanilla
   extract

1–2 teaspoons runny honey
   (optional)
1 apple (optional)

Porridge is a fantastically filling breakfast, especially on a winter morning. Here's a brilliant idea for a dairy-free version. I make it with soya milk but you can experiment with other milks – look out for oat and almond but make sure to buy the unsweetened varieties. If none of these are to hand, you can also make this with skimmed cow's milk or even water.

* * *

1 Put the oats, milk, dates and vanilla extract into a heavy-based saucepan with 300ml water. Bring to the boil over a medium-high heat then reduce the heat to low and simmer, stirring often, for 7–8 minutes until thick and creamy.

2 Meanwhile, if you are using the apple, core and coarsely grate it, leaving the skin on. Stir in most of the apple, and drizzle with honey if you like it a little sweeter.

3 Divide into two bowls, top with the remaining apple if using, and serve.

FLAT MUSHROOMS
WITH WILTED SPINACH AND POACHED EGGS

SERVES

100% mild and light olive
   oil spray
2 sprigs fresh thyme
2 large flat mushrooms,
   stalks removed
pinch of flaked sea salt,
   such as Maldon

freshly ground black
   pepper
2 large handfuls baby
   spinach
2 medium free-range eggs,
   at room temperature

To finish
15g fresh parmesan cheese,
   shaved with a peeler
few fresh thyme leaves

**This is a delicious dish to start the day;
even one that I'd make at lunchtime.
Poaching eggs reveals their true
freshness: old eggs will splay out in the
water whereas the freshest will poach
neatly, so make sure you use ones that
are as fresh as possible. And that's the
secret – they're really not hard to cook!**

★ ★ ★

1 Three-quarter fill a small saucepan
with water and bring to the boil.

2 Place a medium non-stick frying pan
over a medium heat and spray with olive
oil. Add the sprigs of thyme and place
a mushroom, stalk side down, on top
of each. Press a small flat pan lid directly
onto the mushrooms, leaving there
so they have a little weight. Cook for
4 minutes then remove the pan lid
and turn the mushrooms over.

3 Season the just-cooked side
with salt and pepper and cover the
mushrooms with spinach leaves, filling
the pan. Continue to cook uncovered
for a further 4 minutes or until most
of the water has evaporated, now
discard the thyme sprigs.

4 Crack the eggs into the boiling
water and simmer for 2 minutes or
to your liking; remove with a slotted
spoon onto kitchen paper to drain.

5 Serve each mushroom on a warmed
plate, filled with wilted spinach and top
with a poached egg. Season with salt
and freshly ground black pepper and
cover with parmesan shavings and
a few thyme leaves.

SCRAMBLED EGG AND TOMATO
ON RYE TOAST

SERVES

100% mild and light olive
    oil spray
100g vine-ripened cherry
    tomatoes, cut into
    quarters
pinch of flaked sea salt,
    such as Maldon

100g rye bread (2 large
    slices or 4 small slices,
    max 190 calories) or 2
    small seeded pitta breads
2 medium free-range eggs,
    lightly beaten

To serve
Few strands of chives,
    finely chopped (optional)
freshly ground black pepper

Simple ones are always the best!
Tomatoes and soft-cooked scrambled
eggs have a natural affinity that is really
underrated. This is so easy yet delicious
– enjoy it as a lunch or light supper too.
Rye toast is always my first choice for
toast but if you prefer you can have it
inside a toasted seeded pitta. Garnish
with chopped chives if you have them
to hand.

* * *

*For meltingly soft, creamy scrambled egg,
cook gently and take off the heat when it's still
a little undercooked and stir through at the
last minute – you can taste the difference!*

* * *

1 Heat a medium non-stick pan over a
medium heat and spritz with oil. When
hot add the tomatoes and a pinch of salt
flakes; stir. Lower the heat and cook for
about 3 minutes until the tomatoes are
soft and have a little colour.

2 Toast the rye bread or seeded
pitta breads.

3 Increase the heat of the pan a little
and add the beaten eggs to the
tomatoes. Mix once and leave for 1–2
minutes undisturbed – look out for the
egg to be just cooked around the edge
of the pan then remove from the heat
and stir gently until softly scrambled
and just cooked.

4 Place onto the toast or inside split
pitta breads and sprinkle with chives
if using and a few twists of freshly
ground black pepper.

SMOKED SALMON AND SPINACH SPELT PANCAKES

SERVES

For the pancakes
2 tablespoons spelt
   flour
4 heaped tablespoons
   unsweetened natural
   yoghurt (about 4% fat)
1 medium free-range egg
¼ teaspoon bicarbonate
   of soda

1 lemon, finely grated zest
   and wedges to garnish
large handful baby spinach
   leaves, plus small leaves
   to garnish
pinch of flaked sea salt,
   such as Maldon
100% mild and light olive
   oil spray

To finish
100g smoked salmon
2 tablespoons unsweetened
   natural yoghurt (about
   4% fat)
freshly ground black pepper

This is like a giant smoked-salmon-topped blini and great for breakfast, brunch or even lunch. Spelt makes a nice change and has a sweet nutty flavour, but regular flour can be used in its place if you prefer. The pancake is easy to make and cooks quickly but is nonetheless impressive.

* * *

If you don't have time to make the pancakes try toasted spelt bread or even share a wholemeal bagel if you like.

* * *

1 In a medium bowl use a balloon whisk to mix the flour, yoghurt, egg, bicarbonate of soda and most of the lemon zest, reserving a little for garnish. Tear the spinach leaves by hand into small bits and add to the mixture with a pinch of salt. Mix well to combine.

2 Place a wide non-stick frying pan on a medium heat and lightly spray with oil. Spoon the mixture into the pan in two circles and cook for 2–3 minutes each side. Remove and rest the pancakes on a plate for 1 minute.

3 Top each pancake with a few small spinach leaves, then the smoked salmon. Finish off with a tablespoon of yoghurt on each pancake, a sprinkle of lemon zest and some freshly ground black pepper.

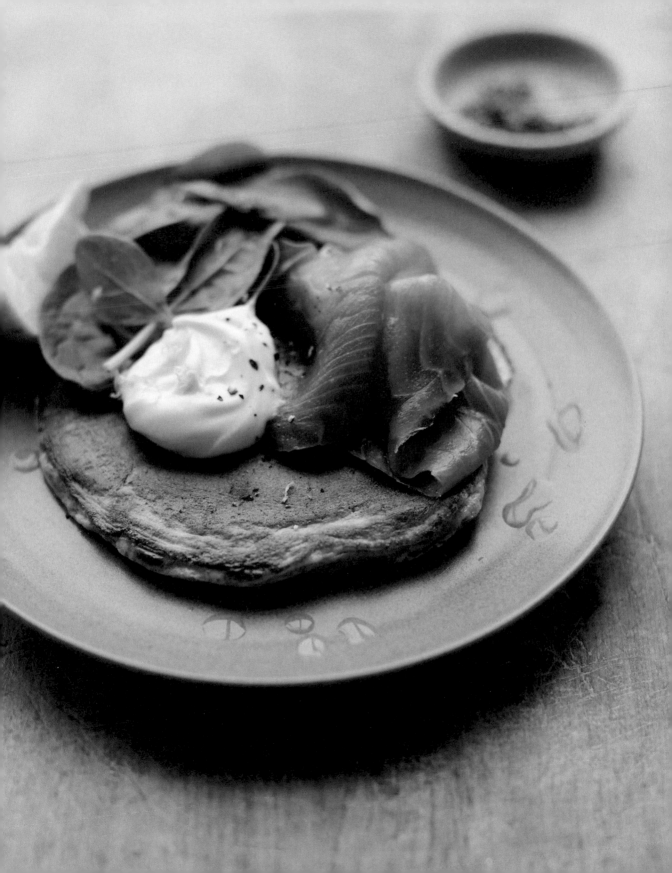

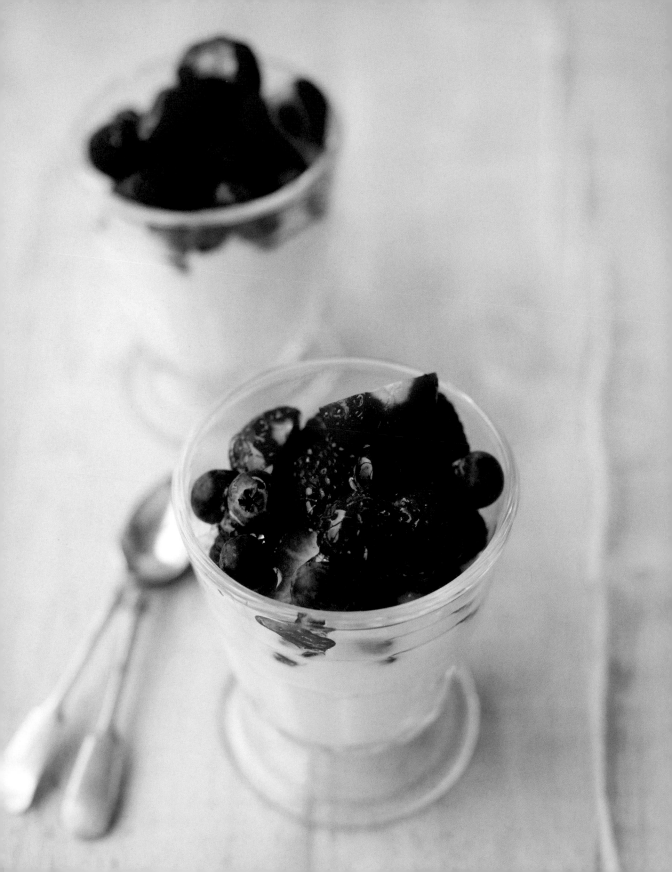

BREAKFAST SUNDAE

SERVES

2

300g unsweetened
natural yoghurt
(about 4% fat)
100g strawberries, cut
into quarters

100g raspberries
100g blueberries
2 tablespoons No-sugar
granola stash from
page 116 (optional)

1 teaspoon runny honey or
agave syrup (optional)

This is simple to make in the morning; ideal when time is short, and the ingredients can be easily halved to make a super-speedy breakfast for one. The good news is there is no need to buy low-fat or fat-free yoghurt – keep to this portion of full-fat yoghurt and enjoy it! This will keep you satisfied through the morning. You could add a tablespoon of granola to each bowl or, if you have a sweet tooth, then by all means add a drizzle of honey – wildflower honey works well with dairy.

1 Layer the ingredients into glass bowls.

2 If using, drizzle with honey or agave syrup, or sprinkle with granola.

* * *

If I have the granola or the honey, I tend to go for a 0% fat greek yoghurt instead.

* * *

* * *

NO-SUGAR GRANOLA STASH

MAKES (PORTIONS)

8

200g jumbo oats
25g pumpkin seeds
25g sunflower seeds
40g almonds in skins,
   roughly chopped

1 teaspoon ground cinnamon
1 tablespoon sunflower oil
1 tablespoon agave syrup
   or maple syrup
1 teaspoon vanilla extract

180ml apple juice,
   freshly pressed not
   from concentrate
60g raisins and/or
   other dried fruit

Shop-bought granolas can be packed with sugar and oil. This is a super-healthy version that I always try and keep a batch of in my cupboard for breakfasts or snacks in a hurry. I love it with fat-free natural yoghurt and a few fresh berries, or with unsweetened almond or oat milk. Sometimes I'll grab a handful straight from the jar to keep me going through a busy afternoon.

* * *

You can try different dried fruits — look out for dried cherries, blueberries, cranberries, apricots or even goji berries.

* * *

1 Preheat a fan oven to 180°C.

2 Line a large baking tray with baking parchment. Toss all the dry ingredients together (apart from the raisins) on the baking tray. In a bowl mix together the sunflower oil, agave syrup and vanilla extract then stir in the apple juice. Pour over the dry ingredients and toss really well to thoroughly distribute the liquid. Spread out to cover the base of the tin and cook in the oven for 30 minutes, stirring every 10 minutes.

3 Leave to cool completely then stir in the dried fruit. Transfer to an airtight container and keep for up to two weeks.

RICOTTA, BANANA AND HONEY
ON RYE TOAST

SERVES

100g rye bread (2 large
  slices or 4 small slices,
  max 190 calories)

60g ricotta
1 large banana, sliced
  diagonally

pinch ground cinnamon
1 teaspoon runny honey

A super-speedy breakfast that packs an indulgent punch while still low on calories. I love rye bread, and always have the pre-sliced loaves in for breakfasts.

* * *

If you have any banana left over you can freeze it in chunks and use it to make gorgeous, thick smoothies straight from the freezer.

* * *

1 Toast the slices of rye bread in a toaster.

2 Spread with the ricotta then top with the sliced banana. Sprinkle with a pinch of cinnamon and drizzle over the honey to serve.

BLUEBERRY AND PISTACHIO BIRCHER

SERVES
2

approx. 100ml apple
   juice, freshly pressed
   not from concentrate
50g porridge oats
   (not jumbo)

1 small apple
2 tablespoons unsweetened
   natural yoghurt
   (about 4% fat)

20g pistachio nut kernels
30g blueberries

Bircher muesli was originally developed by a Swiss doctor to help restore his patients' health. The base is great for all the family as it's soft enough for babies and children to enjoy. The rest of the family can play around with the recipe to include their favourite nuts, seeds and fresh or dried fruits. The oats will provide slow release energy to help ward off hunger throughout the morning. Just one warning – it's easy to get obsessed with!

★ ★ ★

1 Slowly pour apple juice over the oats until it's just visible around the edge then leave to rest for at least 10 minutes or overnight in the fridge.

2 Core and coarsely grate the apple, leaving the skin on. Mix the apple and yoghurt into the oats and top with the nuts and blueberries.

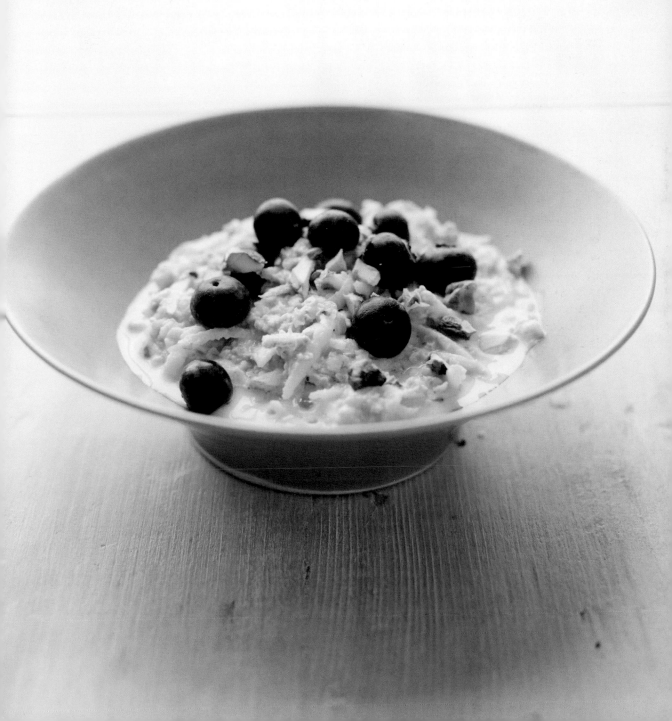

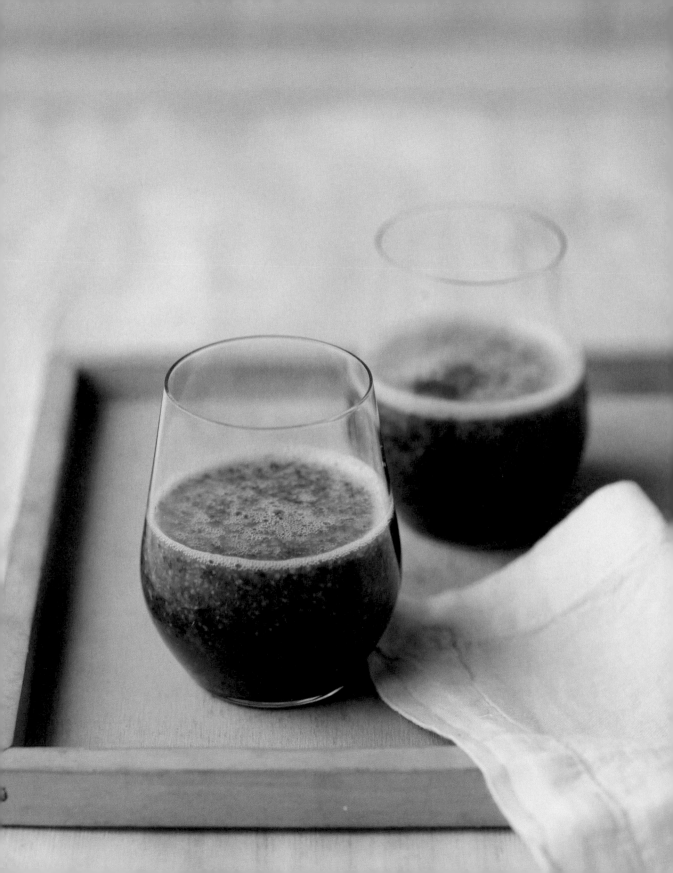

SIMPLE GREEN SMOOTHIE

SERVES

2

100g kale (prepped weight),
stalks removed
25g spinach
2 medium green apples,
skins left on, cored and
roughly chopped

4cm piece ginger, peeled
and roughly chopped
1 tablespoon freshly
squeezed lime juice

400–500ml pure coconut
water, not from
concentrate
2 teaspoons chia seeds
(optional)

Don't be put off by the idea of green smoothies – they're absolutely amazing and I've grown to love them! This is the ultimate healthy snack or breakfast, absolutely packed with green goodness. Coconut water is available in most supermarkets alongside fresh juice; you can replace half the coconut water with water if you prefer. Chia seeds are also becoming more widely available but don't feel you need to add them unless you happen to have some knocking about. Keep all your ingredients in the fridge so the smoothie is nice and cold, and drink it as soon as you can after making it for the maximum health boost.

1 Thoroughly wash the kale leaves in cold water along with the spinach to get rid of any grit. Drain off excess water and put in a blender.

2 Add all the remaining ingredients with 400ml of the coconut water and 1 teaspoon of the chia seeds, if using. Blend thoroughly until smooth. It should be nice and thick, but if it's so thick you can't drink it add the remaining coconut water until you get the desired consistency.

3 Serve straight away, sprinkled with the remaining chia seeds.

* * *

*The smoothie will keep in a thermos flask
for 3–4 hours if you want to take it to
work with you – just give it a gentle stir
or shake before drinking.*

* * *

BERRY AND VANILLA SMOOTHIE

SERVES
2

100g strawberries
100g raspberries
100g blueberries
½ small avocado,
    peeled

2 tablespoons ground
    almonds (optional)
200–250ml apple juice,
    freshly pressed not from
    concentrate (200ml

for fresh berries, more
    for frozen berries)
1 scant teaspoon vanilla
    extract

Berries are widely available frozen with no effect on nutritional value, which makes them not only great to have to hand just when needed but also ideal for the winter months. Avocado adds good fats to this antioxidant-packed smoothie and gives it a creamy texture without adding dairy. Lacing with vanilla extract is also a clever trick to increase the perceived sweetness without adding sugar or honey.

* * *

1 Place all of the ingredients into a blender and blitz until smooth.

2 Pour into two large glasses to serve.

* * *

If you don't have any avocado for this smoothie, replace with a small banana or 2 heaped tablespoons natural unsweetened yoghurt.

* * *

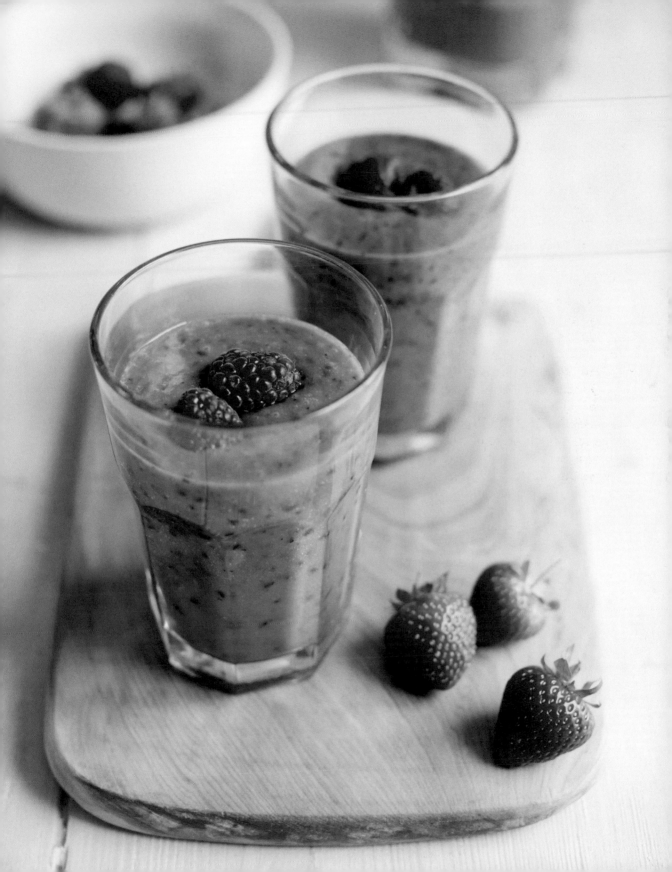

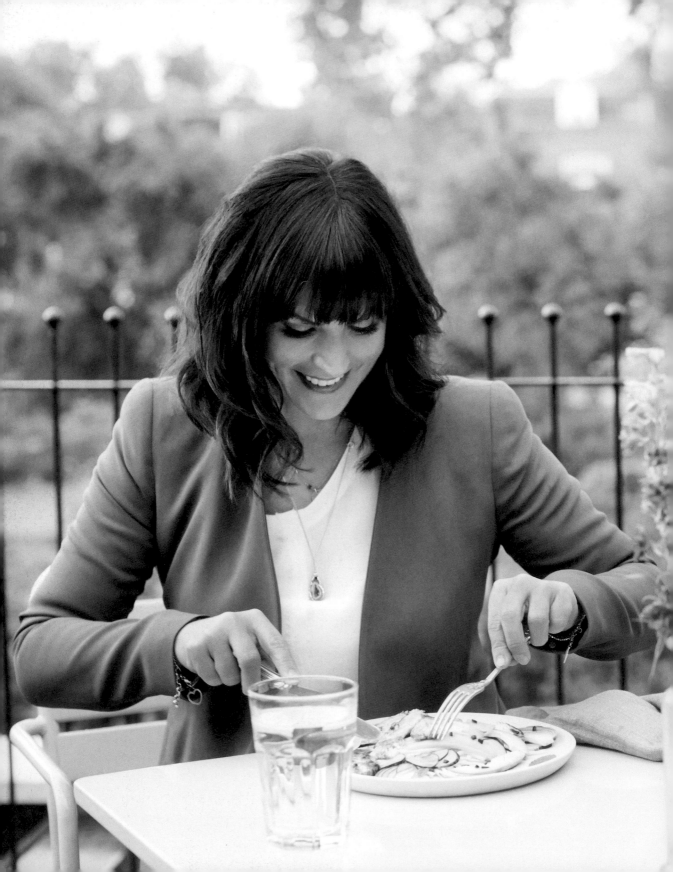

LUNCHES

*Who doesn't love lunch? It's my favourite meal of the day and
I'm never happier than when I can spend it with friends or family.
But sometimes, particularly if you're busy and working in an office,
the temptation is just to grab a sandwich and eat it at your desk.*

*With a little bit of organization and a well-stocked fridge, there's
no reason why we can't enjoy something healthier. All of these lunches
have been created so that they're simple and wholesome, and many
can be easily packed in a pot if needs be. They're also around
500 calories each — more then enough to fill you.*

*If you have no option but to eat out, be sure to try and
buy fresh food that reflects what we have here in the recipes
and stick to the calorie limit where possible.*

TUNA AND WHITE BEAN SALAD

SERVES

1 x 200g tin tuna in olive oil
½ medium red onion,
    finely diced
½ x 400g tin cannellini
    beans, drained and rinsed
½ medium yellow pepper,
    seeds removed,
    finely diced

½ medium orange pepper,
    seeds removed, finely
    diced
150g vine-ripened tomatoes,
    cut into quarters if small
    or eighths if large
small handful fresh coriander,
    tender stalks and leaves

chopped, plus a few
    leaves to garnish
1 small bird's eye chilli, seeds
    removed, finely chopped
pinch of flaked sea salt,
    such as Maldon

This is a bright and nutritionally balanced salad that is really quick to prepare and, although it is great served straight away, it gets better over time so is perfect to be made in the morning and eaten at lunchtime. The salt releases all of the juice from the tomatoes and mixes superbly with the olive oil from the tin of tuna making a seriously good dressing with minimal effort!

★ ★ ★

1 Empty the contents of the tin of tuna, including olive oil, into a large serving bowl.

2 Add the rest of the ingredients, mix thoroughly and season with sea salt flakes.

3 Serve scattered with a few coriander leaves or rest in the refrigerator to garnish and eat later.

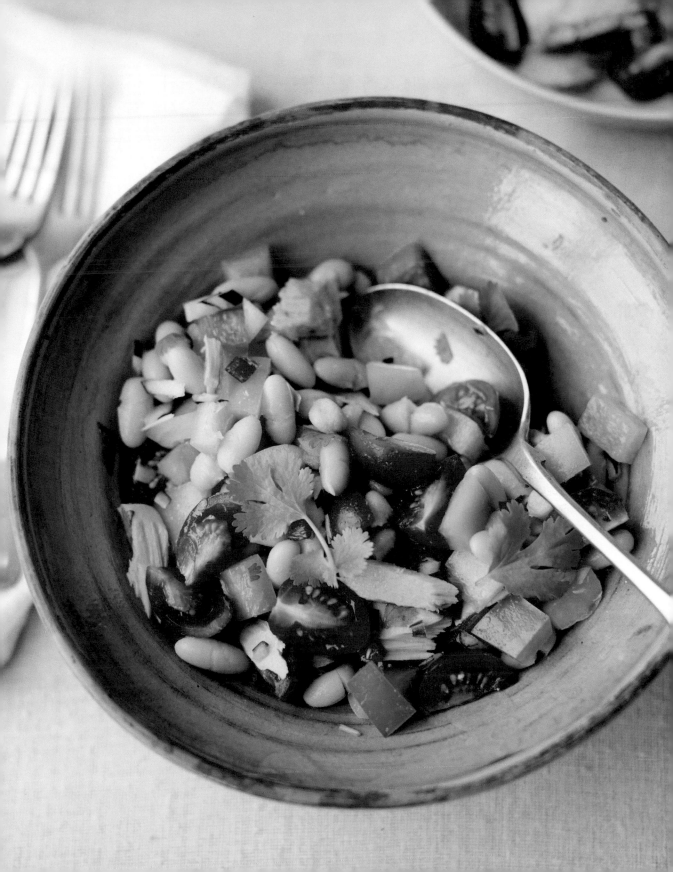

ROASTED VEGETABLE
AND PUY LENTIL SALAD

SERVES

2 red romero peppers,
   seeds removed, cut
   into 4cm chunks
2 small courgettes, halved
   lengthways and cut
   into 4cm chunks
1 medium aubergine,
   cut into 4cm chunks
2 medium vine-ripened
   tomatoes, cut into eighths

1 medium red onion
2 cloves garlic, skins
   left on
100% extra virgin olive
   oil spray
2 tablespoons balsamic
   vinegar
pinch of flaked sea salt,
   such as Maldon
freshly ground black pepper

1 x 400g tin Puy lentils,
   drained and rinsed
large handful fresh herbs
   (any combination of
   flatleaf parsley, basil,
   mint, chervil), leaves
   roughly chopped

I love this veggie-packed lunch that's filling but still less than 500 calories. It is delicious hot or cold and can be kept for at least a day so you can save some for tomorrow's packed lunch. You could hold back a handful of the roast veg and use to stuff a pitta bread or wheat-free wrap with a good handful of rocket for another quick lunch.

* * *

*Use lots of fresh herbs –
more than you might think!*

* * *

1 Preheat a fan oven to 200°C.

2 Tip the pepper, courgette, aubergine, tomato and onion onto a large (preferably non-stick) roasting tin or, to cook them a bit quicker, two smaller trays. Bash the garlic cloves to break the skin, but leave whole, and add to the vegetables. Spray with olive oil then toss together really well so everything is thoroughly coated. Pour over the balsamic vinegar, season with salt and pepper and roast for 25–30 minutes, stirring once or twice. Don't rush the roasting stage – make sure the vegetables are softened and golden-brown at the edges to give a natural sweetness.

3 Mix the drained lentils and fresh herbs together and divide between two plates. Spoon the roasted vegetables on top and serve.

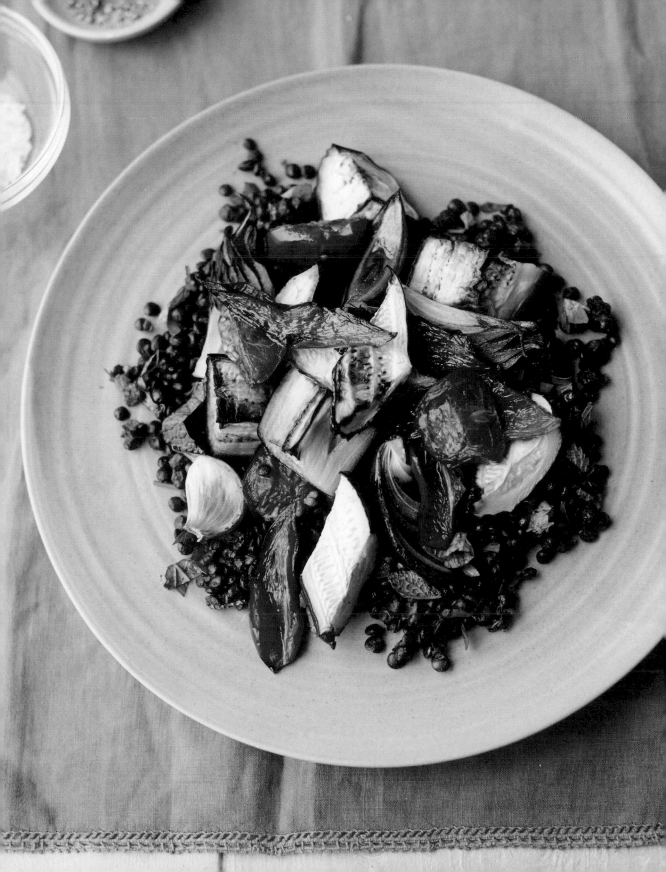

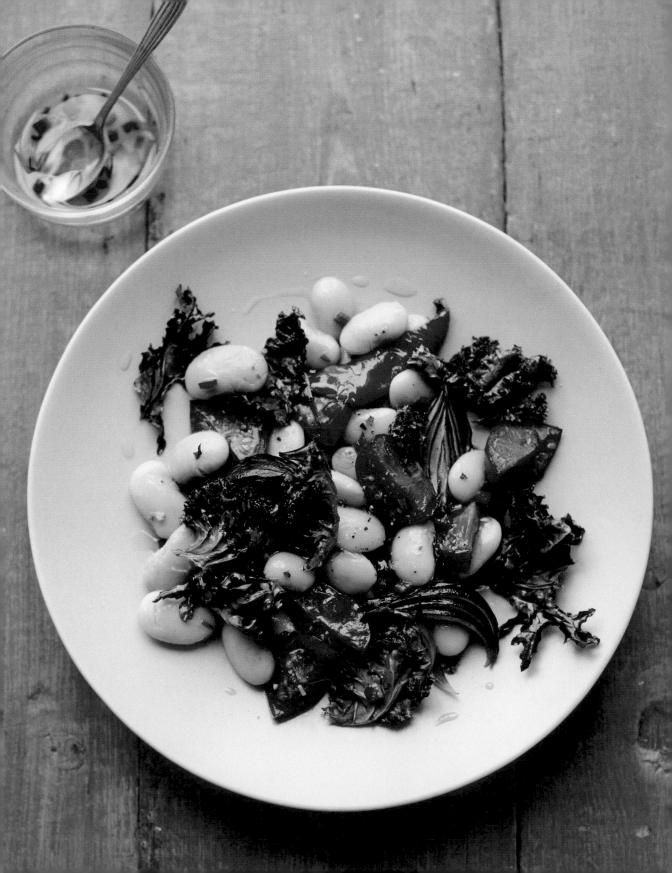

KALE AND ROASTED RED VEG SALAD

For the salad
300g vine-ripened
tomatoes, cut into
quarters if small or
eighths if large
2 red romero peppers,
seeds removed, cut
into 2cm slices
1 medium red onion, cut
into 1cm slices
3 sprigs fresh rosemary,
needles pulled off

100% extra virgin olive
oil spray
pinch of flaked sea salt,
such as Maldon
1 x 400g tin butter
beans, drained
and rinsed

For the kale
100g kale (prepped weight),
stalks removed, washed
and dried

100% extra virgin olive
oil spray
pinch of flaked sea salt,
such as Maldon

For the dressing
1–2 teaspoons extra virgin
olive oil
2 tablespoons freshly
squeezed lime juice
½ mild red chilli, seeds
removed, finely chopped

I like to use a mix of large and cherry tomatoes for this recipe. It looks lovely and gives different textures. The kale goes lovely and crunchy, but be careful not to overcook it as it seems to go from crisp to frazzled in a matter of minutes.

★ ★ ★

You can buy bags of ready-prepared kale in the supermarket. If you're preparing it yourself strip the leaves off the tough stalks, discard the stalks and roughly tear the leaves.

★ ★ ★

1 Preheat a fan oven to 200°C.

2 Tip the tomatoes, peppers and onions onto a large non-stick roasting tray and toss with the rosemary needles, olive oil and some salt. Roast for 20–25 minutes until softened and sticky. Stir in the butter beans and roast for a further 2–3 minutes to heat through.

3 Spray the kale with olive oil and sprinkle with salt. Use your hands to rub the oil into the kale, covering it evenly. Roast for 7–9 minutes until crisp and then remove from the oven.

4 To make the dressing, whisk the oil, lime juice and chopped chilli together.

5 Toss everything together and serve.

SHREDDED CUMIN CHICKEN
WITH MANGO AND CHILLI SALAD

SERVES

2

For the chicken
2 medium free-range
    boneless, skinless
    chicken breasts
    (approx. 300g)
100% mild and light olive
    oil spray
1 teaspoon ground
    cumin
½ teaspoon chilli powder

pinch of flaked sea salt,
    such as Maldon
freshly ground black pepper

For the salad
150g white cabbage,
    core removed
75g radishes, sliced
½ small red onion,
    cut into half moons

½ small ripe mango,
    cut into thin slices
1 red chilli, seeds removed,
    finely chopped
about 10 fresh mint leaves
½ medium avocado, peeled
    and sliced into strips
1 lime

This is a really tasty way to incorporate a rainbow of vegetables into lunch without it feeling too virtuous. Cooking chicken this way makes it soft and juicy, the perfect savoury balance for the sweet spicy salad. For a slight variation, try replacing the cabbage with Chinese leaf.

* * *

1 Place each chicken breast between two sheets of cling film on a chopping board and hit firmly with a wooden rolling pin to flatten to just under 1cm thick (don't worry if holes or tears appear in the chicken).

2 Discard the cling film and place the flattened chicken into a bowl spray lightly with oil and coat well with the spices. Season with salt and pepper.

3 Shred the cabbage very finely with a knife or mandoline, or coarsely grate it. Combine with the other salad ingredients in a bowl and squeeze over the juice of half the lime, cut the remaining half into two wedges to garnish. Mix the lime juice into the salad until the cabbage softens.

4 Heat a medium non-stick frying pan over a medium heat and add the chicken, cooking for 4 minutes. Turn the chicken over and turn the heat to low. Cover with a lid that stops the steam escaping and continue to cook on the lowest heat for 5 more minutes.

5 In the pan use two forks to shred the chicken along the grain, soaking up any juice. Be careful not to scratch the pan!

6 Divide the salad between two plates and top with the chicken and wedges of lime to serve.

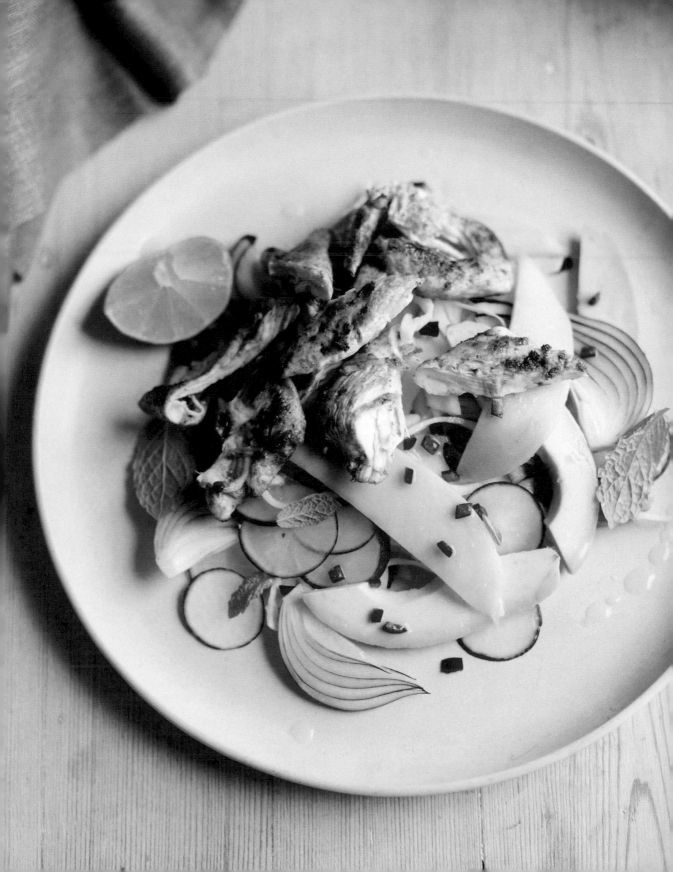

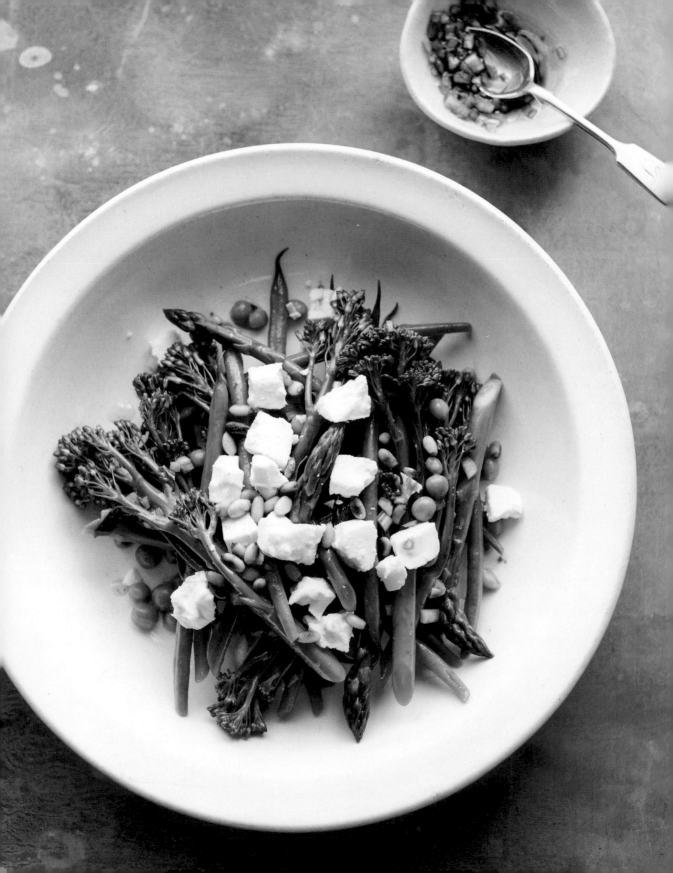

HOT GREEN BEAN AND FETA SALAD

SERVES

2

For the salad
20g pine nuts
150g green beans, trimmed
150g tenderstem broccoli
and/or asparagus,
trimmed
100g frozen peas
60g feta cheese, crumbled

For the dressing
1 shallot, finely chopped
(optional)
1 tablespoon balsamic
vinegar
1 small orange, finely
grated zest and
2 tablespoons juice

1 tablespoon extra virgin
olive oil
pinch of flaked sea salt,
such as Maldon
freshly ground black pepper

I love this crunchy green salad, full of interesting textures and surprise flavours. It's one of my favourite lunches when I haven't got much time to cook; any leftovers are great cold as a packed lunch.

* * *

The dressing will keep in the fridge for at least three days.

* * *

1 Heat a frying pan over a medium heat, add the pine nuts and cook for 3–4 minutes, shaking the pan every now and again, until toasted. Tip onto a plate to cool. Alternatively toast in a fan oven at 180°C for 2–3 minutes.

2 For the dressing, whisk together all the ingredients, or tip into a jam jar, screw the lid on tightly and shake well.

3 Bring a large pan of salted water to the boil, add the green beans and broccoli or asparagus and boil for 3 minutes, then add the peas and cook for a further minute. The veg should be just tender but still with some crunch. Drain thoroughly, return to the pan and toss through the dressing.

4 Transfer to two bowls. Scatter with the feta and pine nuts and serve.

TOASTED CASHEW AND RED CHILLI BEEF

SERVES
2

250g stir-fry beef steak strips or frying steak, cut into thin strips
1 tablespoon oyster sauce
100% mild and light olive oil spray
1 lime, finely grated zest and half the juice
1 tablespoon mirin (Japanese rice wine)

25g whole natural cashew nuts
1 fat clove garlic, finely chopped
2cm piece ginger, peeled and finely chopped
½ medium pepper, seeds removed, cut into thin strips (any colour)
1 medium carrot, cut into matchsticks

1 medium head pak choi, washed and sliced
1 large red chilli, seeds removed, diagonally sliced
2 thick spring onions, outer leaves and tops removed, cut into chunks diagonally

---

Although this meal is low-carb there is plenty of protein to fill you up and the zingy flavours will leave you really satisfied, plus it's so quick to make! Make sure all of the prep is done before you start and don't leave the pan once you start cooking; the vegetables want to be bright and colourful and they are easy to overcook.

* * *

1 Coat the beef strips in the oyster sauce and a few sprays of oil and set aside.

2 Mix the lime zest, juice and mirin together in a small bowl as a dressing. Set aside.

3 Heat a wide non-stick frying pan or dry wok over a medium heat and add the cashew nuts. Turn so they colour all over, – it will take about 2 minutes – taking care not to let them burn. Remove the nuts from the pan and set aside.

4 Turn the heat to high and spray the pan with oil. Once the oil is hot add the garlic and ginger tossing for 30 seconds to infuse the oil.

5 Add the steak strips and fry for 1 minute stirring often. Add the vegetables and fry for a further 2 minutes, again stirring often.

6 Pour the lime dressing into the side of the pan and let it bubble. Mix in the red chilli. Remove from the heat and stir in the toasted cashew nuts.

7 Divide between two warm bowls and serve.

* * *

Give the vegetables a really good pat dry with kitchen paper as you prepare them so that they don't steam in the pan.

* * *

VIETNAMESE PRAWN OMELETTE

For the pak choi
2 heads pak choi
2 teaspoons dark soy sauce
1 clove garlic, finely
    chopped (optional)
1 teaspoon sunflower oil
    (optional)

For the omelette
4 medium free-range eggs
handful fresh coriander,
    tender stalks and
    leaves chopped

2 teaspoons nam pla
    (Thai fish sauce) or
    dark soy sauce
1½ teaspoons sunflower
    or vegetable or
    groundnut oil
6 spring onions, outer leaves
    and tops removed, green
    and white parts sliced
1 mild red chilli, seeds
    removed, finely chopped,
    plus extra to garnish
    if you like

1 fat clove garlic,
    finely chopped
200g raw prawns,
    defrosted if frozen,
    roughly chopped
about 10 fresh mint leaves

This makes a great super-quick dinner.
I like to have it with wilted pak choi but
to make it even easier serve it with a
salad of baby spinach and thinly sliced
cucumber dressed with a splash of wine
vinegar. I make one large omelette to
save time, but they look lovely made as
individual omelettes in a smaller pan.

* * *

1 Cut the pak choi lengthways into
quarters. Arrange in a steamer over
a pan of boiling water and steam for
5 minutes until just tender. (Or you can
boil them for 3–4 minutes.) Drizzle over
the soy sauce. If using the garlic, heat
the oil in a small pan over a medium
heat, add the garlic and fry for 2 minutes
until sizzling and golden. Spoon over
the pak choi. Keep warm.

2 Add the eggs, coriander, nam pla
and 2 tablespoons water to a bowl
and beat lightly.

3 Heat ½ teaspoon of the oil in a large
non-stick frying pan over a medium-high
heat (make sure you use a non-stick pan
otherwise the omelette will stick). Add
the spring onions, chilli and garlic and
fry for 1 minute.

CONTINUED OVERLEAF

VIETNAMESE PRAWN OMELETTE

CONTINUED

4 Increase the heat to high, add the prawns and cook for 1–2 minutes until the prawns turn pink and any excess water evaporates. Transfer to a bowl.

5 Wipe around the pan with a piece of kitchen paper and add the remaining oil. Place over a medium-high heat then pour in the eggs and cook for 1 minute until they are just starting to set on the bottom. Scatter over the prawn mixture and cook for a further 2–3 minutes until the eggs have almost set. To finish cooking the top of the omelette you can either fold the omelette in half and cook for a further 2 minutes, or pop it under a preheated medium-high grill for 1–2 minutes.

6 Turn out the omelette and scatter with torn mint leaves. You can garnish with some thinly sliced red chilli if you like the heat. Serve with the steamed pak choi alongside.

★ ★ ★

Use frozen prawns so you can take out what you need and defrost them in the fridge for about three hours before you need them. I prefer to use small Atlantic or Canadian prawns but farmed king prawns will work too.

★ ★ ★

QUICK COCONUT CURRY

SERVES
2

200ml coconut milk
3 tablespoons Thai
    curry paste
50g tenderstem broccoli,
    cut into smaller florets
½ medium red pepper,
    seeds removed, cut
    into thin strips

200g microwaveable
    brown rice
250g skinless and
    boneless cod fillet
    (or other firm white
    fish), cut into bite-
    size chunks

small handful fresh
    coriander, tender stalks
    and leaves (optional)

If you need a satisfying supper in a hurry then this is a great option. Supermarkets these days stock a wide variety of curry pastes, many of them are exceptional quality with all natural ingredients. Once you find a favourite paste it will become a great midweek supper. All of the vegetables cook in the sauce to keep all the nutrients, feel free to swap and change for your favourites. Don't be put off choosing brown rice because you are short of time! This recipe uses microwavable pouches, widely available these days, and perfect to serve with this quick curry.

* * *

1 Place a non-stick frying pan over a medium heat; add 2 tablespoons coconut milk and the curry paste and stir. Heat until bubbling – this will only take about 30 seconds – then add the vegetables. Toss to coat them then add the remaining coconut milk.

2 Heat the rice as per the packet instructions.

3 Once the curry is bubbling, gently lower in the fish and cover with a lid to stop the steam escaping. Allow to bubble for a further 3 minutes.

4 Serve in warmed bowls with the rice and scattered with coriander leaves if you have them to hand. Season if necessary.

WHOLEGRAIN GREEN RISOTTO

SERVES

2

For the green purée
100g baby spinach
small handful fresh
    coriander and/or flatleaf
    parsley, tender stalks and
    leaves chopped
½ mild green chilli,
    seeds removed,
    roughly chopped

2 heaped teaspoons
    vegetable bouillon powder

For the risotto
100% mild and light olive
    oil spray
8 spring onions, outer leaves
    and tops removed, green
    and white parts sliced

160g brown basmati rice
100g frozen peas, defrosted
100g green beans, trimmed
    and cut into 4cm pieces
1 tablespoon freshly
    squeezed lime juice
15g freshly grated parmesan
freshly ground black pepper

**This is my super wholesome version
of a classic risotto. The brown rice takes
a bit longer to cook but it's worth it
and will keep you fuller for longer.**

* * *

1 For the purée, chuck the spinach,
herbs, chilli and bouillon powder into
a blender. Add 250ml water and blitz
to a purée.

2 Spray a large, heavy-based (preferably
non-stick) frying pan or saucepan with
olive oil and place over a medium heat.
Add the spring onions and fry for 2–3
minutes until just softened. Stir in the
rice and fry for one minute then add the
green purée plus another 350ml water.
Bring to a simmer, stir once, cover the
pan and simmer over a medium heat
for 25 minutes.

3 After 25 minutes of cooking stir the
rice and check the texture – it should
be just tender and most of the liquid
absorbed; add a splash more boiling
water if needed and cook for a few
more minutes. Scatter the peas and
beans over the rice, cover with the lid
and cook for a further 5 minutes.

4 Use a fork to gently fold the beans
and peas into the rice along with the
lime juice and half the parmesan.

5 Scatter over the remaining parmesan
and some freshly ground black pepper
and serve.

* * *

*Defrost peas in a flash by
tipping them into a sieve and pouring
boiling water over them.*

* * *

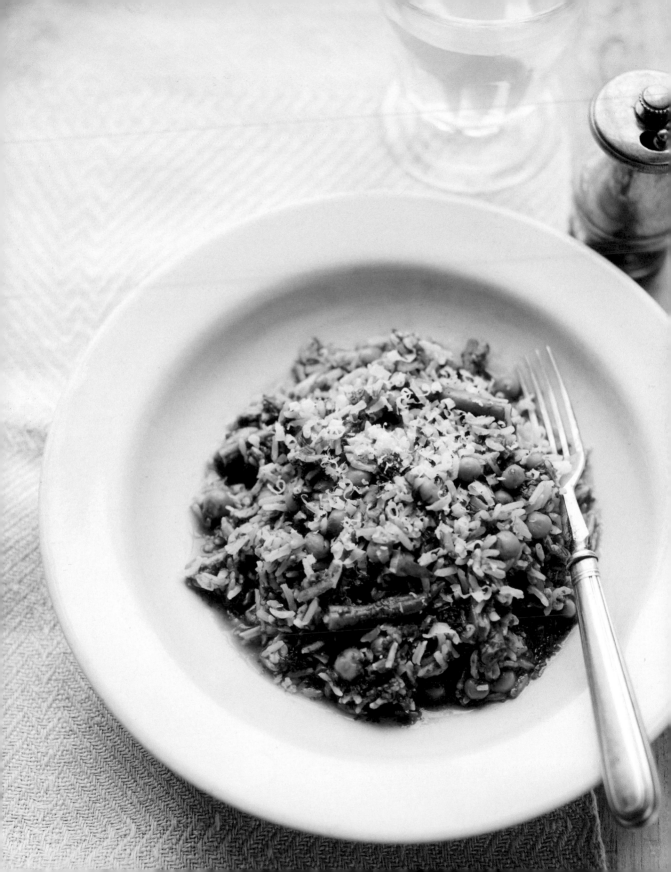

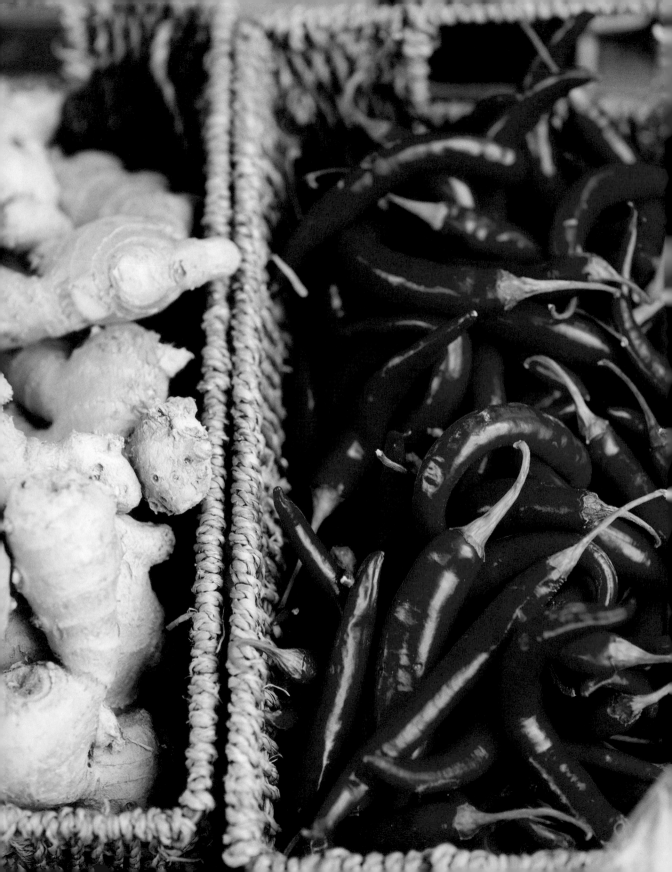

JAPANESE CRUNCHY VEG NOODLES
WITH TOFU

SERVES

2

For the noodles
150g soba noodles (also
    called buckwheat noodles)
1 tablespoon dark soy sauce
1 tablespoon mirin
    (Japanese rice wine)
1 teaspoon toasted sesame oil
150g radishes, sliced
100g sugar snap peas or
    mangetout, trimmed

1 medium courgette,
    halved lengthways
    and thinly sliced on
    the diagonal

For the tofu
4cm piece ginger, peeled
    and finely grated
1 fat clove garlic, finely
    chopped

½ red chilli, seeds removed,
    finely chopped
2 teaspoons dark soy sauce
100% mild and light olive
    oil spray
200g firm tofu, cut into
    1cm slices
about 10 fresh mint leaves

**This tofu is packed full of flavour and
tastes amazing with the Japanese-style
noodles. I like to leave the veggies raw
because I love the crunch and freshness,
but if you prefer your vegetables
cooked, then simply replace the
radishes with red pepper and steam all
the veg for a couple of minutes before
tossing them through the noodles.**

* * *

1 Bring a large pan of water to the boil,
add the soba noodles and cook for 5
minutes until just tender but not mushy
(or as per packet instructions) – don't
overcook or they will break up. Use
a large pan as the water can rise up
as the noodles cook.

2 Drain and rinse the noodles. Return to
the pan and toss through the remaining
noodle ingredients. Set aside.

3 In a small bowl mix together the
ginger, garlic, red chilli and soy sauce.

4 Spray a non-stick pan with the olive
oil and place over a medium-high heat.
Dab the tofu dry with kitchen towel then
place in the pan. Fry for 2–3 minutes on
each side, until the slices have a golden-
brown crust.

5 Transfer to warm serving plates and
spoon the ginger-garlic soy sauce over
the tofu. Scatter with torn fresh mint leaves
and serve with the noodles alongside.

* * *

*The really good soba noodles are made with
100 per cent buckwheat and are gluten-free. Some are
a mix of buckwheat and regular wheat. You could
replace the soba noodles with brown rice noodles
or wholewheat noodles, just be sure each portion
of noodles is no more than 280 calories.*

* * *

CHILLI PRAWN CAKES
WITH RIBBON VEGETABLES AND SPICY HUMMUS

SERVES

2

For the prawn cakes
small handful fresh coriander,
    tender stalks and leaves
1 spring onion, outer leaves
    and top removed
1 small red bird's eye chilli,
    seeds removed

1 teaspoon oyster sauce
230g raw king prawns,
    defrosted if frozen
100% mild and light olive
    oil spray

To finish
1 large carrot, cut into
    ribbons using a peeler
1 large courgette, cut into
    ribbons using a peeler
2 portions of Spicy hummus
    from page 212

Raw king prawns are great to keep in
the freezer and use when there is little
time to shop. Buy them frozen and
when ready, cook from frozen or defrost
quickly at room temperature. This
recipe uses defrosted prawns to make
a healthy delicious hot lunch for two or
a fantastic impromptu plate of nibbles.

★ ★ ★

*Instead of using the spicy hummus,
you could stir a chopped chilli into a bought
pot of plain hummus.*

★ ★ ★

1 Into a mini chopper or food processor
add the coriander, spring onion, chilli
and oyster sauce and blitz until chopped
finely. Add half of the prawns and
blitz again until smooth, then add the
remaining prawns and pulse until
coarsely combined.

2 Divide the mixture in half and with
your hands shape three patties from
each half making six in total.

3 Spritz a large non-stick pan with
the oil on a high heat and fry the prawn
cakes for 3 minutes each side. Turn the
heat to low and cover the pan with a
lid that stops the steam escaping for
2 more minutes.

4 Remove the prawn cakes onto warmed
plates to rest. Increase the heat on the
pan and add the vegetables, stirring to
coat in the juice. Cook for 1 minute. Serve
alongside the cakes with a portion of
the spicy hummus from page 212.

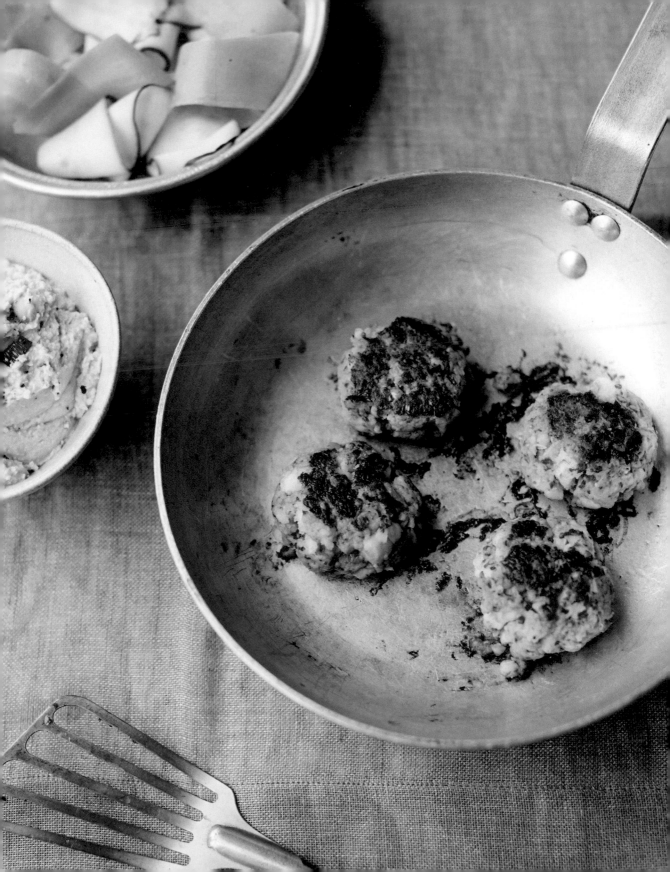

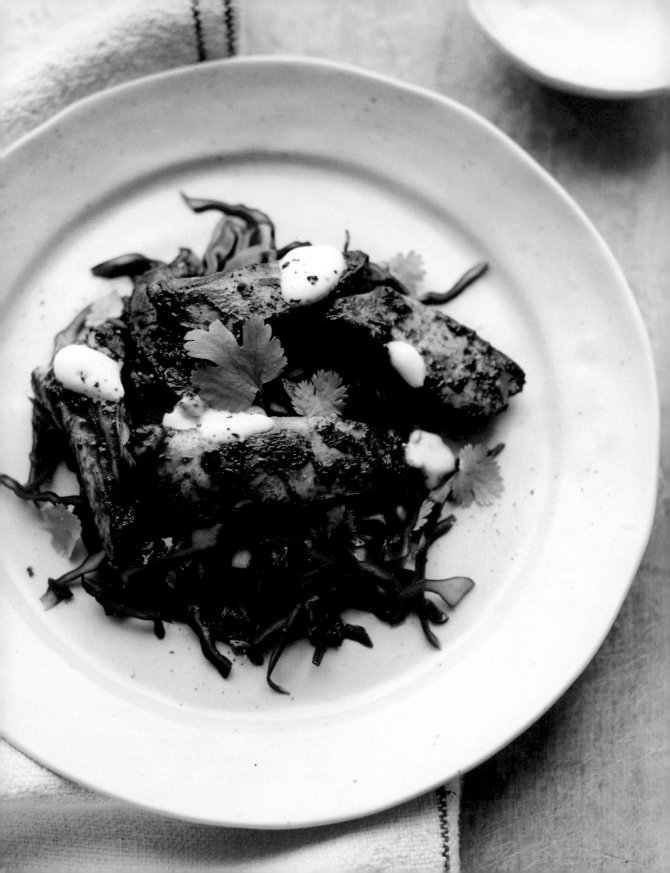

CHIPOTLE CHICKEN
WITH QUICK PICKLED CABBAGE

SERVES

100g red cabbage,
    core removed
1 heaped tablespoon
    brown sugar
125ml white malt vinegar
1½ teaspoons salt
300g free-range skinless
    chicken mini fillets

1½ tablespoons chipotle
    paste
100% mild and light olive
    oil spray
2 heaped tablespoons
    unsweetened natural
    yoghurt (about 4% fat)

pinch of flaked sea salt,
    such as Maldon
freshly ground black pepper
small handful fresh
    coriander, tender stalks
    and leaves

Chipotle paste is now available in most supermarkets and is a fantastically versatile store cupboard ingredient; from stirring into a chilli to making a dressing for roasted vegetables. It is made from smoke-dried jalapeño peppers and instantly delivers a deep smoky heat. Paired with the pickled cabbage and yoghurt this dish will certainly wake up your taste buds and makes a great hot lunch or quick supper.

★ ★ ★

1 Shred the cabbage very finely using a food processor, mandoline or very sharp knife, and tip into a wide shallow bowl.

2 Mix together the sugar, vinegar and salt until dissolved. Pour over the cabbage and mix well. Set aside, mixing occasionally.

3 Coat the chicken with the chipotle paste.

4 Spritz a wide shallow frying pan with a small amount of oil. Place over a medium heat and, when hot, add the chicken and cook for 3–4 minutes each side.

5 Season the yoghurt with sea salt flakes and pepper.

6 Drain the cabbage (this removes most of the sugar) and mix in the coriander leaves.

7 Transfer the pickled cabbage to two plates. Serve with the chicken on top and dress with the yoghurt.

MEXICAN STREET FOOD TACOS
WITH QUICK CORIANDER SALSA

SERVES

2

For the pink onions
½ medium red onion,
    thinly sliced
1 tablespoon freshly
    squeezed lime juice
pinch of flaked sea salt,
    such as Maldon

For the beans
100% mild and light olive
    oil spray
½ medium red onion,
    thinly sliced
1 heaped teaspoon
    ground cumin

1 x 400g tin black beans
    or pinto beans, drained
½ teaspoon vegetable
    bouillon powder
½ mild red chilli, seeds
    removed, finely chopped
small handful fresh
    coriander, tender stalks
    and leaves chopped
pinch of flaked sea salt,
    such as Maldon
freshly ground black
    pepper

For the salsa
2 medium vine-ripened
    tomatoes, finely chopped
½ mild red chilli, seeds
    removed, finely chopped
1 tablespoon freshly
    squeezed lime juice
small handful fresh
    coriander, tender stalks
    and leaves chopped
pinch of flaked sea salt,
    such as Maldon

To finish
4 ready-made corn tacos

**These are a fab lunch and only take 10
minutes if you do a spot of multi tasking
and make the salsa while the beans are
cooking. Instead of the corn tacos you
can use wholegrain or wheat-free wraps.**

∗ ∗ ∗

1 Preheat a fan oven to 180°C.

2 Toss the onion with the lime juice
and salt in a shallow bowl and set aside.

3 Spray a non-stick frying pan lightly
with olive oil and place over a medium-
high heat. Add the onions and fry
for 5 minutes until softened and
turning golden.

4 Stir in the cumin and fry for 30
seconds then stir in the beans, bouillon
and 75ml water. Simmer vigorously
for 3–4 minutes then mash a few of
the beans against the side of the pan.
Stir through the red chilli and coriander
and season with salt and black pepper.

5 While the beans are simmering,
toss the salsa ingredients together.
Pop the tacos in the oven to reheat
according to packet instructions.

6 Drain any excess liquid off the
onions and stir this into the beans.

7 Fill the tacos with the warm black
beans followed by the coriander salsa.
Scatter over the pink onions and serve.

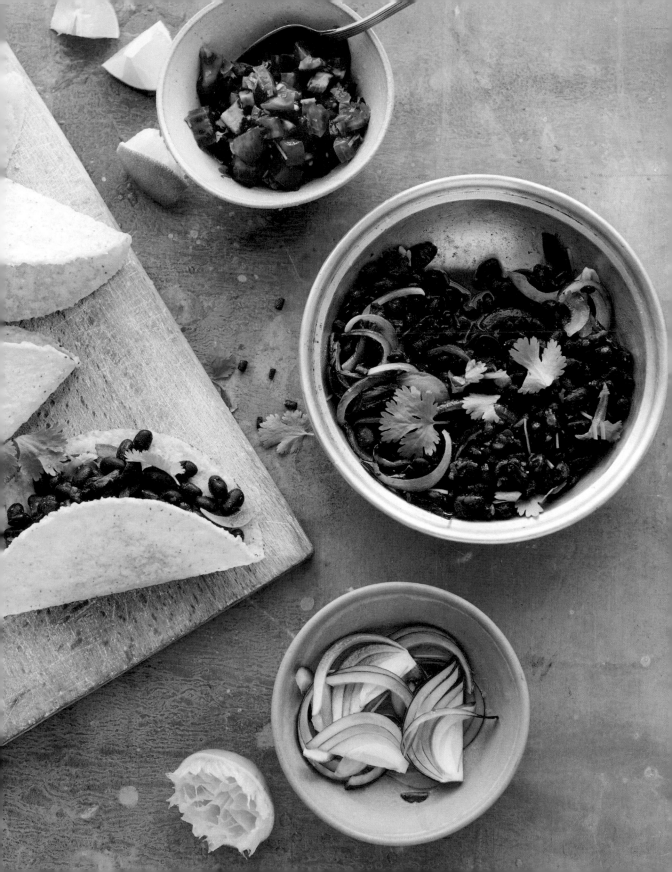

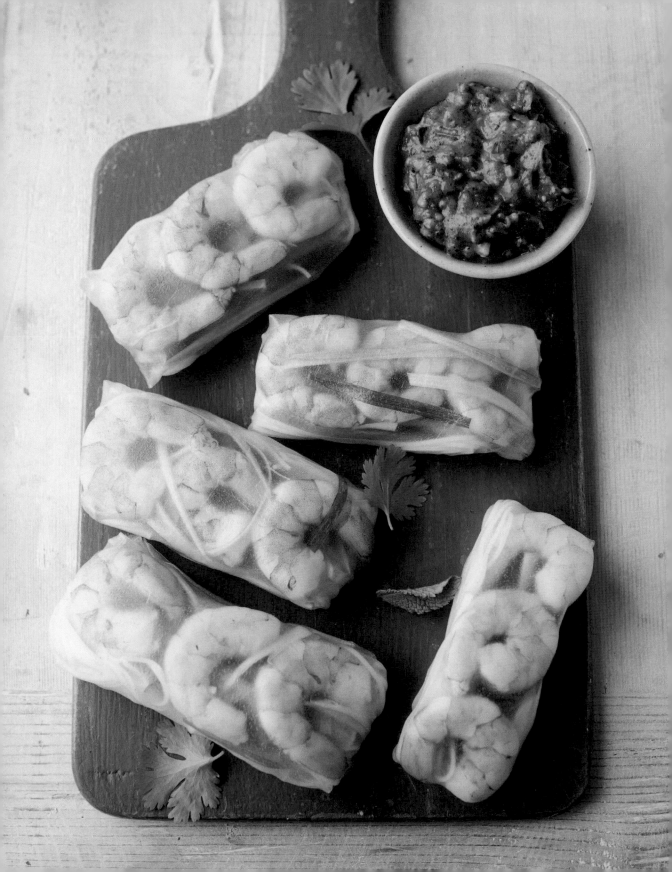

VIETNAMESE SUMMER ROLLS
WITH SPICY PEANUT DIPPING SAUCE

For the dipping sauce
3 tablespoons unsweetened
   crunchy peanut butter
1½ teaspoons nam pla
   (Thai fish sauce)
1 large lime, finely grated
   zest and juice
2 teaspoons runny honey
1½ teaspoons Japanese
   rice vinegar
1 red chilli, seeds removed,
   finely chopped

For the salad
1 large carrot, grated or cut
   into very fine matchsticks
3 spring onions, outer leaves
   and tops removed, finely
   shredded lengthways
small handful fresh
   coriander, tender stalks
   and leaves torn, plus
   a few leaves to garnish
½ lime, juice only
1 teaspoon nam pla
   (Thai fish sauce)

To finish
20g dried instant vermicelli
   rice noodles
½ teaspoon toasted
   sesame oil
250ml vegetable stock
   (choose very good
   quality organic stock
   cubes)
18 raw king prawns,
   fresh or frozen
6 rice paper wrappers
small handful fresh
   coriander and/or mint,
   tender stalks and leaves

I have to confess that I'm slightly obsessed with these – spicy dipping sauce and transparent little parcels that just about show you their delicious fillings. They are adaptable to whatever you have in the fridge or just what you fancy. Some food for thought: cucumber, pepper, radish, beansprouts, mangetout, lettuce, avocado, mint, Thai basil, chives. The wrappers are made of rice and are available in bigger supermarkets often called spring roll wrappers, but if you can't get hold of them you could do this in little gem lettuce cups, or wrapped in an iceberg lettuce leaf. They are quick to prepare and great for a lunch on the move.

1 Combine all the dipping sauce ingredients into a small bowl and mix thoroughly. Set aside.

2 Combine the carrot, spring onions and coriander in a bowl and dress with the lime juice and fish sauce. Mix well and set aside.

3 Cover the instant noodles in boiling water for 2 minutes then drain and plunge into cold water. Drain well and place on kitchen paper, then tip into a clean bowl and coat in the sesame oil, set aside.

CONTINUED OVERLEAF

* * *

VIETNAMESE SUMMER ROLLS
WITH SPICY PEANUT DIPPING SAUCE
CONTINUED

4 Place the vegetable stock in a small pan and bring to a gentle bubble then add the prawns until they turn pink. This will take approximately 2–3 minutes from chilled or 4–5 minutes from frozen. Reserving the stock, remove the prawns with a slotted spoon and set aside to cool.

5 Tip the poaching stock into a shallow bowl that is as wide as the rice paper wrappers and leave to cool a little.

6 Once the poaching stock is just warm take a wrapper and hold at 9 o'clock with one hand and 3 o'clock with the other and lean the top away from you. Working very quickly dip the bottom into the stock so that it reaches the centre and rotate the wrapper clockwise so it is wet all over, then lay flat. Don't be tempted to keep dipping the wrapper as it will continue to rehydrate while flat.

7 Line up three prawns horizontally in the centre of a wrapper and top with salad then noodles.

8 Fold the bottom away from you over the filling then fold in each side. Pick up the final edge and roll to finish.

9 Sprinkle the fresh herbs over, and serve three rolls per person, with the spicy peanut dipping sauce.

* * *

You could present these as a salad by combining all of the salad ingredients and drizzling over the dressing then covering with one softened wrapper per person. Garnish with herbs and edible flowers.

* * *

SMOKED CHICKEN
AND GRAPEFRUIT CUPS

20g pine nuts
160g whole smoked
   chicken breast
1 red grapefruit, segments
   and 1 tablespoon of juice

1 teaspoon mild olive oil
½ medium avocado,
   peeled and finely diced
3 little gem lettuce hearts,
   16 leaves separated,

tiny leaves in the centre
discarded

These are a fabulous alternative to a sandwich. Smoked chicken breast works brilliantly but if you can't get hold of it a plain cooked chicken breast will work just as well.

★ ★ ★

To segment the grapefruit use a serrated knife to cut the top and bottom off the grapefruit then sit it flat on one end and use the knife to work top to bottom removing all the skin from the sides. Slide the knife along each of the membranes to remove each segment. Squeeze the pith over a bowl to collect the juice.

★ ★ ★

1 Heat a small non-stick pan and add the pine nuts to toast for about 3 minutes mixing once to turn them – take care as these can easily burn. Switch off the heat and set aside in the pan.

2 Using your hands, shred the chicken breast into small strips and place into a medium bowl.

3 Break each of the grapefruit segments into three or four pieces and add to the chicken. Then add the grapefruit juice, olive oil, avocado and toasted pine nuts. Mix well to combine.

4 Fill each lettuce leaf with the mixture and serve eight cups per person.

SCANDI BEETROOT AND SMOKED SALMON MINI FRITTATA

For the frittata
100% mild and light olive
    oil spray
2 medium free-range eggs
small handful watercress,
    finely chopped
1 teaspoon chopped
    dill fronds
pinch of flaked sea salt,
    such as Maldon
freshly ground black pepper

For the dressing
1 tablespoon freshly
    squeezed lemon juice
1 teaspoon wholegrain
    mustard
1 teaspoon mild olive oil
1 teaspoon chopped
    dill fronds
½ teaspoon runny honey

To finish
30g watercress
1 medium raw beetroot,
    peeled and grated
100g hot smoked salmon,
    flaked into large chunks

I used to serve this on a slice of rye and then one day I had the genius idea of serving it on a mini frittata for extra protein. It only takes five minutes to cook, but if you're too busy you can swap it for a thin slice of rye (just be sure the rye bread is no more than 115 calories). Served on the frittata this makes a great weekend lunch or brunch.

* * *

For a really cute touch, use a mini frying pan (about 8cm in diameter) for perfect mini frittatas.

* * *

1 Heat a small non-stick frying pan sprayed with a little oil. Lightly beat the eggs with the watercress, dill and salt and pepper. Pour half into the frying pan and fold in the edges as it cooks to create a rough circle. Cook for 2–3 minutes then flip over and cook for a further minute until golden and cooked through. Repeat with the other half.

2 For the Scandi dressing, whisk the mustard into the lemon juice then whisk in the remaining ingredients. Loosen with 2 tablespoons of water if necessary.

3 Mix the watercress, beetroot and salmon together in a bowl and drizzle over the dressing. Divide between the two frittatas and serve.

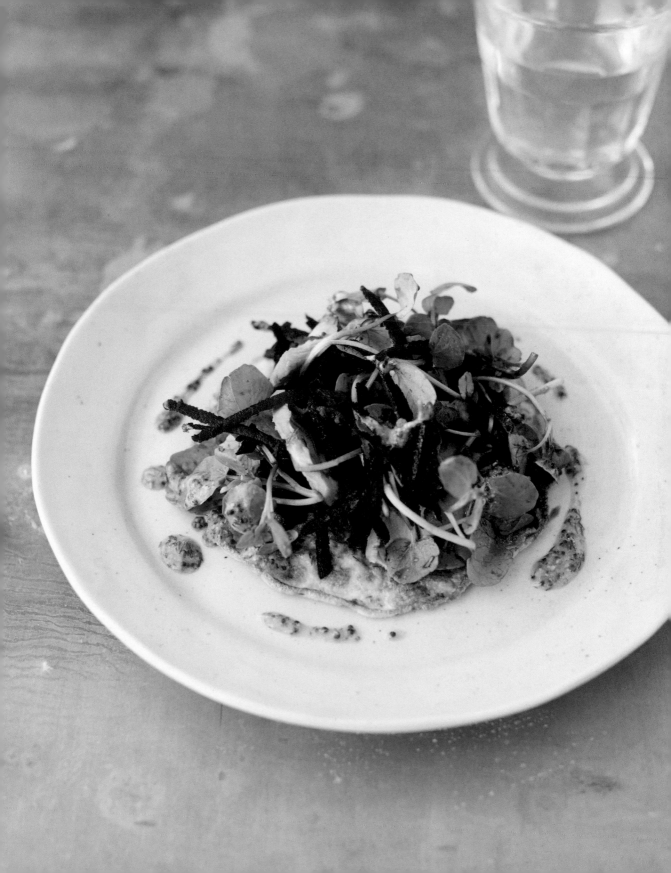

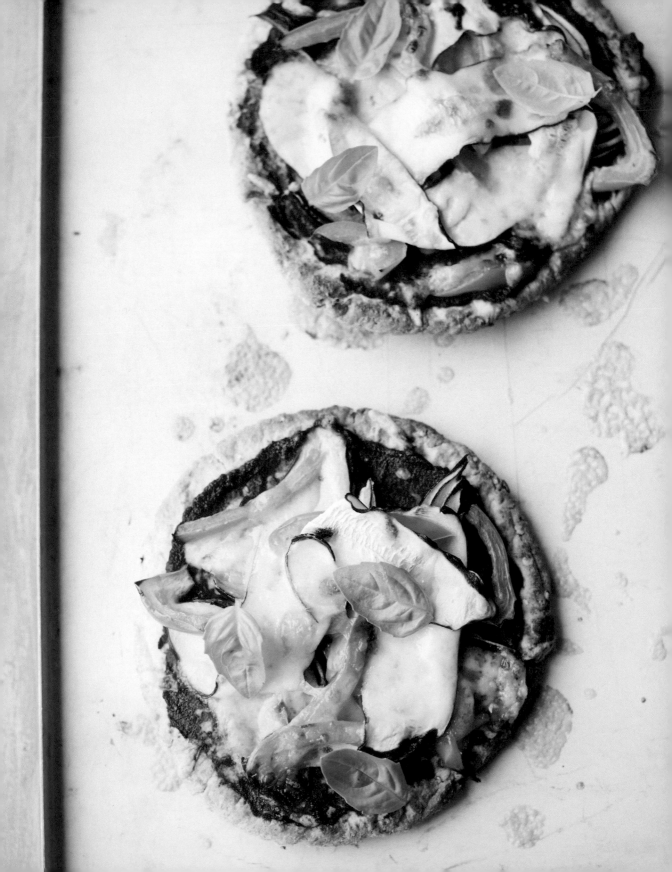

FLATBREAD PIZZAS

2 seeded tortilla or pitta
1 tablespoon tomato purée
1 small red onion,
    finely sliced

½ medium orange pepper,
    seeds removed, sliced
½ small courgette, cut into
    ribbons using a peeler

40g low-fat cheddar cheese
about 10 fresh basil leaves

These are a great weekend lunch to rustle up for all the family, served with a green salad – it's really easy to double-up the quantities. Alternatively, cut each pizza into wedges and serve as a snack. If you're eating it with children, let them choose their favourite toppings or use up what is in the fridge. It's so simple they could probably make it themselves.

★ ★ ★

1 Preheat a fan oven to 180°C.

2 Spread each tortilla with tomato purée, top with the rest of the ingredients finishing with cheese.

3 Bake on a baking tray for around 10 minutes or until the cheese is golden.

4 Garnish with basil leaves and serve.

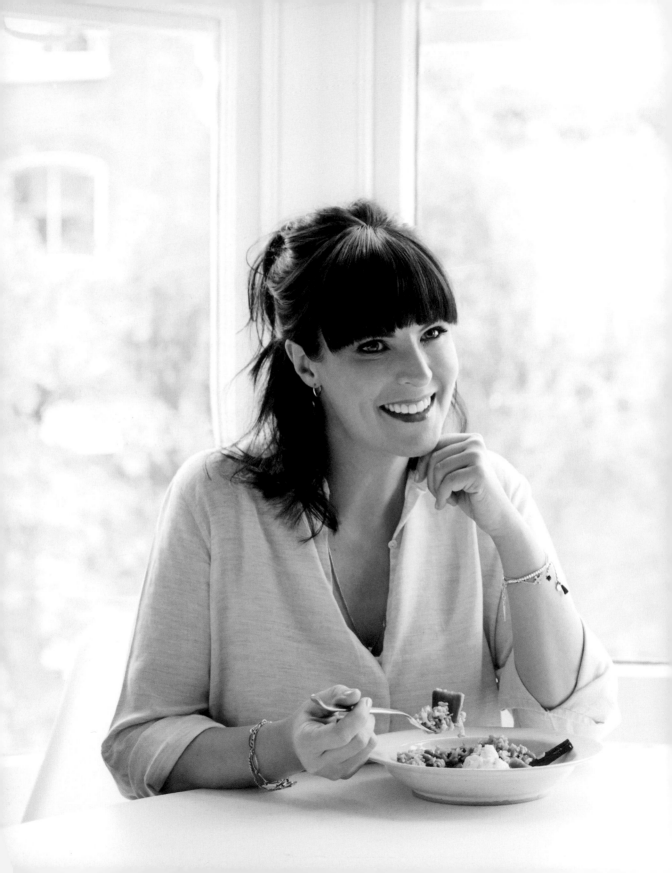

DINNERS

There are fewer things in life more lovely than sitting around a table with the people you cherish and enjoying a home-cooked dinner together. It's a chance to gossip, laugh and reflect on your day.

Making food is an expression of love. Making healthy, mindful food is also an acknowledgment that you care about what you eat. These wholesome, nutritious suppers are designed to be enjoyed by everyone – whether you're on your own, with a loved one or feeding the whole gang.

And what's more – they're only 500 calories per portion. Who said dieting was boring?

STEAMED YOGHURT CHICKEN
AND CUMIN RICE WITH SPICY TOMATO SALAD

SERVES

For the chicken and rice
300g free-range skinless
    chicken mini fillets, cut
    in half lengthways
5 tablespoons unsweetened
    natural yoghurt (about
    4% fat)
2 tablespoons extra hot
    Indian curry paste
½ small red onion,
    finely chopped
½ teaspoon whole cumin
    seeds
100g white pure basmati
    rice

For the salad
150g vine-ripened
    tomatoes, cut into
    quarters if small
    or eighths if large
small handful fresh
    coriander, tender stalks
    and leaves chopped
1 spring onion, outer
    leaves and top removed,
    green and white parts
    finely chopped
1 small red bird's eye chilli,
    seeds removed,
    finely chopped

pinch of flaked sea salt,
    such as Maldon

To finish
2 tablespoons unsweetened
    natural yoghurt (about
    4% fat) (optional)

**If this is healthy eating, bring it on!
Those eating with you won't even realize
there is a health kick happening as this
is so satisfying. There will easily be
second helpings and you will make
it again and again.**

* * *

1 Mix the chicken with the yoghurt and
curry paste. Set aside.

2 In a wide shallow non-stick frying pan
add the onion, cumin, rice and 280ml
water. Mix once, set over a high heat and
boil rapidly uncovered until the water
disappears and it begins to crackle,
turn the heat to the lowest setting.

3 Spread the chicken and yoghurt
mixture over the surface of the rice in
one layer, covering with a large pan lid
so the steam cannot escape. Continue to
cook on the lowest heat for 12 minutes,
or until the chicken is thoroughly
cooked.

4 Meanwhile combine the tomatoes,
coriander, spring onion, chilli and salt
in a medium bowl to make the salad.

5 Serve the rice and yoghurt chicken
on warm plates with the tomato salad
and an extra dollop of yoghurt.

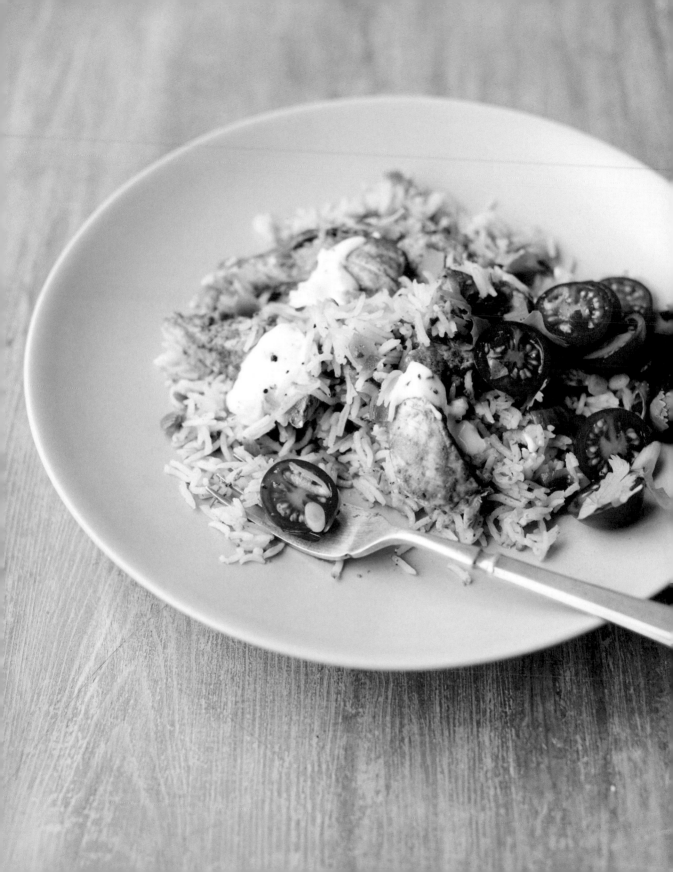

MY FAVOURITE RAGU
WITH SPELT PASTA

SERVES

4

1 tablespoon mild olive oil
100g smoked back bacon
　(about 3–4 rashers),
　excess fat trimmed off,
　cut into thin strips
1 medium onion, finely
　chopped
2 sticks celery, finely
　chopped
2 medium carrots, finely
　diced or grated

2 bay leaves
3 sprigs fresh rosemary
400g beef mince (10% fat)
1 tablespoon balsamic
　vinegar
1 heaped tablespoon
　tomato purée
2 teaspoons vegetable
　bouillon powder
1 x 400g tin chopped
　tomatoes

pinch of flaked sea salt,
　such as Maldon
freshly ground black pepper
50g wholegrain spelt pasta
　per portion (uncooked
　weight), cooked
　according to packet
　instructions
large handful fresh parsley,
　tender stalks and leaves
　chopped

I swear this is as good as any Italian Mama would make. The real secret is the long, slow cooking, so please don't rush it. It freezes brilliantly so I make a batch and freeze it in individual portions for a quick dinner at the end of a busy day. You can use wholegrain spelt pasta, rice pasta or wholewheat pasta.

* * *

1 Heat the oil in a large non-stick lidded frying pan or flameproof casserole over a medium-high heat. Add the bacon and fry for 3 minutes then stir in the onion, celery, carrots, bay leaves and rosemary sprigs. Fry for 10 minutes until softened.

2 Add the beef mince and cook, stirring occasionally to break up any lumps, for 5 minutes until any excess water has boiled off and the mince is starting to brown.

3 Stir in the balsamic vinegar and a couple of tablespoons of water and let it bubble, scraping any browned bits off the bottom of the pan with a wooden spoon. Stir in the tomato purée, vegetable bouillon and tin of tomatoes. Fill the empty tin with cold water and add this to the pan too.

4 Once it starts to bubble, reduce the heat to low, cover with a lid and simmer for 45 minutes to an hour, stirring occasionally and adding a splash of boiling water if it looks dry. Season, to taste with salt and freshly ground black pepper.

5 To serve you can either add the cooked pasta to the ragu and stir it all together, or spoon the ragu on top of the pasta in serving bowls. Top with the chopped parsley.

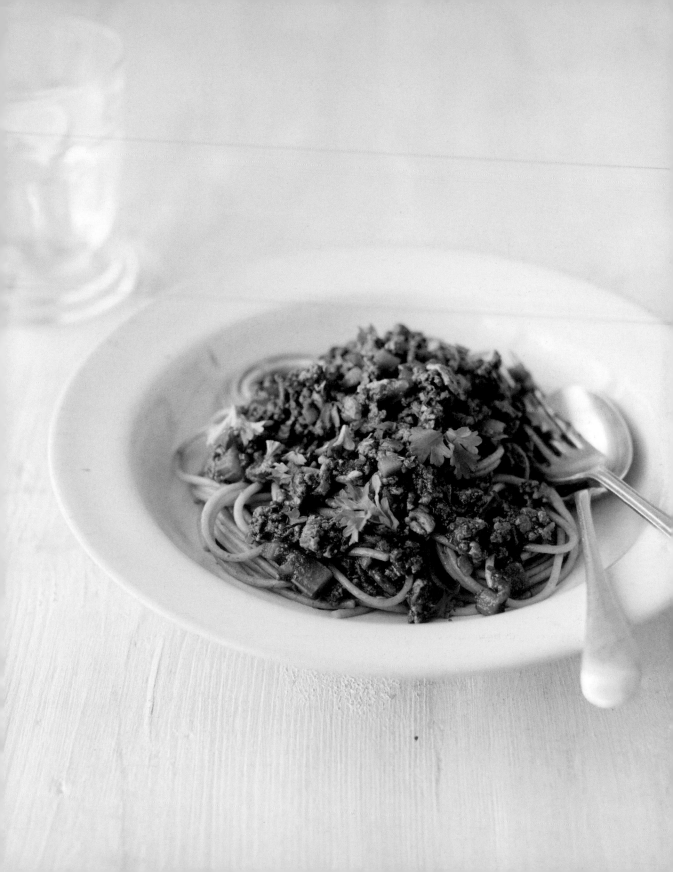

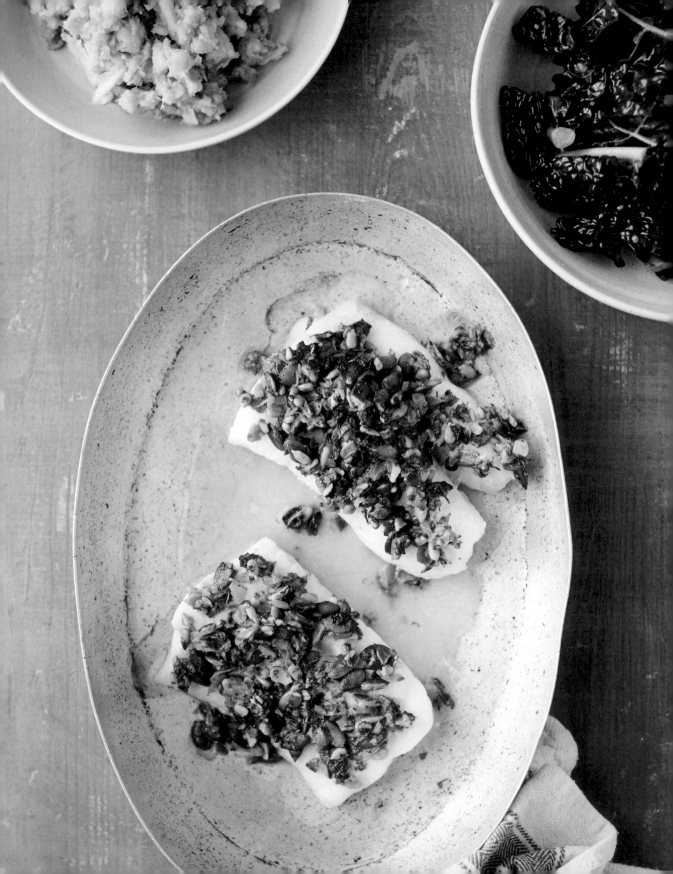

ROAST COD WITH HERBY SEED CRUST
AND CURRIED PARSNIP MASH

SERVES

For the parsnips
1 teaspoon mild olive oil
400g parsnips, peeled and
    cut into 2cm chunks
2 teaspoons mild curry
    powder
1 teaspoon vegetable
    bouillon powder

For the cod
20g pumpkin seeds
10g sunflower seeds
large handful fresh parsley,
    tender stalks and leaves
large handful fresh
    coriander, tender stalks
    and leaves
½ mild green chilli, seeds
    removed, roughly chopped

1 teaspoon mild or extra
    virgin olive oil
pinch of flaked sea salt,
    such as Maldon
1 lime, finely grated zest
    and juice
2 x 200g boneless cod
    loin fillets, skin left on

It might seem like a lot of herbs in the seed crust but trust me, be generous, it tastes amazing! You can use any firm-fleshed white fish for this, or even salmon. Try and buy sustainable fish if you can – ask at the fish counter or check the labelling. Serve it with steamed or boiled greens such as savoy cabbage, spring greens or kale.

* * *

1 Preheat a fan oven to 180°C.

2 Heat the olive oil in a large non-stick saucepan, add the parsnips and curry powder and fry for 2–3 minutes. Pour over 300ml boiling water and stir in the vegetable bouillon. Bring to the boil then cover the pan, lower the heat to medium and cook for 20–25 minutes until completely tender and most of the liquid has been absorbed.

3 Use a potato masher to mash to a smooth consistency, adding a splash of boiling water if needed (you're looking for the consistency of soft mashed potato).

4 While the parsnips are cooking, tip all the ingredients for the cod, apart from the fish itself and half the lime juice, into a mini food processor and blitz to a rough paste (or roughly chop everything using a large, sharp knife). Place the cod in a non-stick roasting tin, spread the paste all over the fish and roast for 12–14 minutes.

5 Squeeze the remaining lime over the cod and serve with the curried parsnip mash on the side.

VEGGIE TWO-BEAN CHILLI
WITH APPLE AND LIME SALSA

SERVES

For the chilli
1 teaspoon olive oil
1 medium red onion, sliced
2 cloves garlic, sliced
1 medium carrot, grated
1½ teaspoons ground cumin
½–1 teaspoon chilli powder
    or paprika, according
    to how hot you like it
heaped ½ teaspoon ground
    cinnamon
1 heaped teaspoon vegetable
    bouillon powder

1 x 680g jar tomato passata
1 medium courgette,
    cut into 1cm chunks
2 medium red, orange or
    yellow peppers or romero
    peppers, seeds removed,
    roughly chopped
1 x 400g tin kidney beans,
    drained and rinsed
1 x 400g tin cannellini
    beans, drained and rinsed

For the salsa
1 apple
1 lime, finely grated zest
    and juice
1 small red onion, finely
    chopped
large handful fresh
    coriander, tender stalks
    and leaves chopped

To finish
2 tablespoons unsweetened
    natural low-fat yoghurt
    (almost 4% fat) (optional)

This is a great one-pot dish – super filling and packed with veggies. You can alternate the beans – try butter beans, chickpeas, cannellini beans or pinto beans too. These quantities shared between two make for a really hearty meal, so if you prefer you could divide it into three, and freeze the third portion to defrost on a day when you need something really quick.

* * *

1 Heat the olive oil in a large non-stick saucepan or flameproof casserole over a medium heat. Add the onions and fry for 5 minutes until just golden, then stir in the garlic and carrot and fry for a further 3 minutes.

2 Stir in the ground spices and fry for 30 seconds, then add 200ml of boiling water, the bouillon powder, passata, courgette, peppers and drained beans. Simmer uncovered over a low-medium heat for 30 minutes, stirring every few minutes and adding a splash of water if it looks too dry at any point.

3 Meanwhile core and coarsely grate the apple, leaving the skin on. Immediately toss the apple with the lime juice to prevent it turning brown. Add the lime zest, red onion and coriander and set aside.

4 Spoon the chilli into warm serving bowls, top with the salsa and a couple of spoonfuls of yoghurt, if using.

HOT ROAST VEGETABLE CURRY

SERVES

2

½ teaspoon ground cumin
1 teaspoon hot curry powder
pinch of flaked sea salt,
    such as Maldon
1 medium aubergine,
    cut into 2cm chunks
200g cauliflower, broken
    into small florets
1 small red onion, sliced
    into rings
2 banana (escallion) shallots,
    quartered lengthways

100% mild and light olive
    oil spray
2 cloves garlic, finely
    chopped
3cm piece ginger, peeled
    and cut into matchsticks
½ teaspoon turmeric
½ teaspoon whole cumin
    seeds
1 tablespoon tomato purée
2 red bird's eye chillies,
    finely sliced

1 x 230g tin chopped
    tomatoes
50g frozen peas
large handful baby
    spinach leaves
3 tablespoons unsweetened
    natural yoghurt
    (about 4% fat)

This is a rich and fiery tomato-based
curry with smoky roasted vegetables.
Meat eaters won't miss meat, plus it
doesn't even need rice or potatoes
to make it satisfying and thoroughly
enjoyable; top with crispy onion rings
and a little yoghurt to temper the heat.

* * *

1 Preheat a fan oven to 200°C.

2 In a small bowl mix together the
cumin, half of the curry powder and
the salt. Set aside.

3 In sections, place the aubergine and
cauliflower onto one large non-stick
baking tray and the red onion slices and
banana shallots onto a second non-stick
baking tray. Spray all with olive oil then
sprinkle all but the shallots with the
cumin, curry powder and salt. Toss each
section well to coat and roast for 25–30
minutes until dark in colour.

CONTINUED OVERLEAF

HOT ROAST VEGETABLE CURRY

CONTINUED

4 Meanwhile, place the garlic and ginger in a medium non-stick pan and spray with oil. Place over a medium heat and sizzle for 1 minute then turn the heat to the lowest setting and cook for 10 minutes without adding any colour.

5 Add a few more sprays of oil and add the turmeric, cumin seeds and remaining curry powder and mix; cook for 3 minutes, then add the tomato purée and red chilli and turn up the heat. Once sizzling add the tin of tomatoes. Fill the empty tin with water to rinse it round and then add to the pan. Cover and simmer for 10 minutes stirring occasionally.

6 When the roasted vegetables are ready set the red onion rings aside for garnish and mix the remaining vegetables into the sauce along with the frozen peas and spinach leaves. Cover and heat through for 3 minutes.

7 Mix through and check the seasoning adding salt if required. Serve in warmed bowls topped with the crispy onion rings and yoghurt.

★ ★ ★

If you prefer a milder dish you can of course reduce the heat by halving or removing the red chillies!

★ ★ ★

ULTIMATE VEGGIE BURGER

SERVES

For the burger
200g sweet potato, skin
    left on, roughly chopped
1 teaspoon olive oil
1 small red onion, finely
    chopped
100g dark mushrooms
    (e.g. Portabellini),
    chopped
1 small courgette, grated
1 small carrot, grated
1 mild red or green
    chilli, seeds removed,
    finely chopped

1 fat clove garlic, finely
    chopped
1 heaped teaspoon
    ground cumin
½ x 400g tin black beans,
    drained and rinsed
1½ tablespoons dark soy
    sauce
1 tablespoon balsamic vinegar
20g raisins
large handful fresh
    coriander, tender stalks
    and leaves chopped
freshly ground black pepper

For the salsa
2 large vine-ripened
    tomatoes, roughly
    chopped
handful fresh coriander
    and/or mint leaves,
    tender stalks and
    leaves chopped
1 teaspoon freshly squeezed
    lime juice
freshly ground black pepper
pinch of flaked sea salt,
    such as Maldon

Loads of veggies make these moist and
tasty burgers stand out from the veggie
burger crowd. Kids love them too – you
can divide the mixture into four and
make smaller burgers if you prefer;
they'll only need 10–15 minutes in the
oven. In winter I have it with a pile of
steamed kale, and in summer I'll go
for a green salad.

* * *

1 Preheat a fan oven to 180°C.

2 Boil the sweet potato in a pan of salted
water for 15 minutes until tender. Drain
thoroughly then mash roughly with a fork.

3 While the potato is cooking, heat
the oil in a non-stick frying pan over a
medium-high heat, add the onions and
fry for 2 minutes. Add the mushrooms
and fry for 5 minutes, stirring often, until
any excess water has evaporated and
they are browning at the edges.

4 Stir in the courgette, carrot, chilli
and garlic and fry for a further 5 minutes
until the vegetables are just softened,
adding splashes of water if they start
to catch.

CONTINUED OVERLEAF

ULTIMATE VEGGIE BURGER

CONTINUED

5 Stir in the ground cumin followed by the black beans, soy sauce and balsamic vinegar. Bubble for a minute or two until all excess liquid has evaporated, then turn off the heat and roughly mash the beans using a potato masher – you want roughly half mashed and half left whole. Stir in the mashed sweet potato, raisins and coriander. Taste the mixture and season with freshly ground black pepper and a little salt if needed (although it should be salty enough from the soy sauce).

6 Let the mixture cool enough to handle, then shape into two large burgers. Place on a non-stick baking tray and cook in the oven for 20 minutes until heated through.

7 While the burgers are cooking, toss together the salsa ingredients. Serve alongside the burgers.

★ ★ ★

The burgers can be chilled in the fridge for up to 24 hours before cooking.

★ ★ ★

SPANISH-STYLE FISH PIE

SERVES

2

2 teaspoons mayonnaise
(optional)
2 cloves garlic, finely
chopped
300g small waxy potatoes
(e.g. Charlotte), cut into
2cm chunks
100% mild and light olive
oil spray

1 teaspoon sweet smoked
paprika
pinch of flaked sea salt,
such as Maldon
1 small red onion, finely
chopped
50g cooking chorizo,
skins removed, cut into
bite-size chunks

1 x 400g tin chopped
tomatoes
250g skinless and boneless
cod fillets, cut into
bite-size chunks
60g tenderstem broccoli,
cut into smaller florets
freshly ground black
pepper

**This is a gutsy satisfying fish dish with
all the strong flavours of Spain and a
delicious 'patatas bravas' style topping
easily assembled at the last minute.**

* * *

1 Preheat a fan oven to 200°C.

2 If using, mix the mayonnaise with
a teaspoon of water and a tiny pinch
of garlic. Set aside.

3 Place the potato chunks into a medium
bowl and spritz with oil. Add half of the
smoked paprika and a pinch of salt, toss
well and spread out onto a non-stick
baking tray and roast in the oven for
20 minutes.

4 Meanwhile, into a medium non-stick
pan add the red onion, remaining garlic
and paprika, chorizo, a pinch of salt and
a few sprays of oil. Set over a low-medium
heat and cook for about 5 minutes
stirring frequently until lightly coloured.

5 Add the tomatoes and bring to the boil
then simmer uncovered over the lowest
heat for 10 minutes, stirring occasionally.

6 Check the seasoning and add a little
more salt if necessary. Increase the
heat to medium then add the cod and
broccoli and stir; cover with a lid for
3 minutes so the fish is just cooked
and the broccoli is bright green.

7 Transfer the mixture into a pie dish
and scatter with the roasted potatoes;
drizzle with the garlic mayonnaise,
if using, and a twist of freshly ground
black pepper.

LEAN ASIAN BEEF BURGER
WITH SHREDDED SALAD

SERVES

2

For the burger
250g lean beef mince
(5% fat)
1 stick lemongrass, tough
leaves removed, tender
middle finely chopped
1 teaspoon nam pla
(Thai fish sauce)
50g roasted red pepper
(bought in a jar)
1 small clove garlic,
finely chopped
small handful fresh
coriander, tender stalks
and leaves finely chopped

freshly ground black pepper
100% mild and light olive
oil spray

For the dressing
2 tablespoons unsweetened
crunchy peanut butter
1 teaspoon nam pla (Thai
fish sauce)
1 lime, finely grated zest and
juice
1 teaspoon runny honey
1 teaspoon Japanese rice
vinegar

For the salad
½ medium cucumber, cut
in half lengthways, soft
middle removed with a
spoon, firm flesh shredded
finely lengthways
3 spring onions, outer leaves
and tops removed, halved
and finely shredded
lengthways
about 10 fresh coriander
stalks, halved
1 fresh red bird's eye chilli,
seeds removed, finely
sliced lengthways

**The Asian twist on this burger means
a bun would just be inappropriate;
salad works perfectly while the peanut
dressing makes this very satisfying.
Increase the quantities to feed more but
cook carefully to keep the burger moist.**

★ ★ ★

1 Into a large bowl add all the burger
ingredients except the oil and combine
thoroughly by hand. Divide the mixture
into two and shape each half into two
wide flat burgers. Set aside.

2 For the dressing combine all of
the ingredients into a small bowl
and mix thoroughly.

3 Combine the salad ingredients
in a medium bowl.

4 Spritz a medium non-stick frying
pan with a few sprays of oil, place over
a medium heat and add the burgers.
Cook for 3 minutes each side, disturbing
at little as possible as pushing and
prodding will cause moisture to escape.
Switch off the heat and cover the pan to
allow the burgers to rest for one minute.

5 Divide the salad between two plates
and spoon over the dressing. Top with
the burger and enjoy!

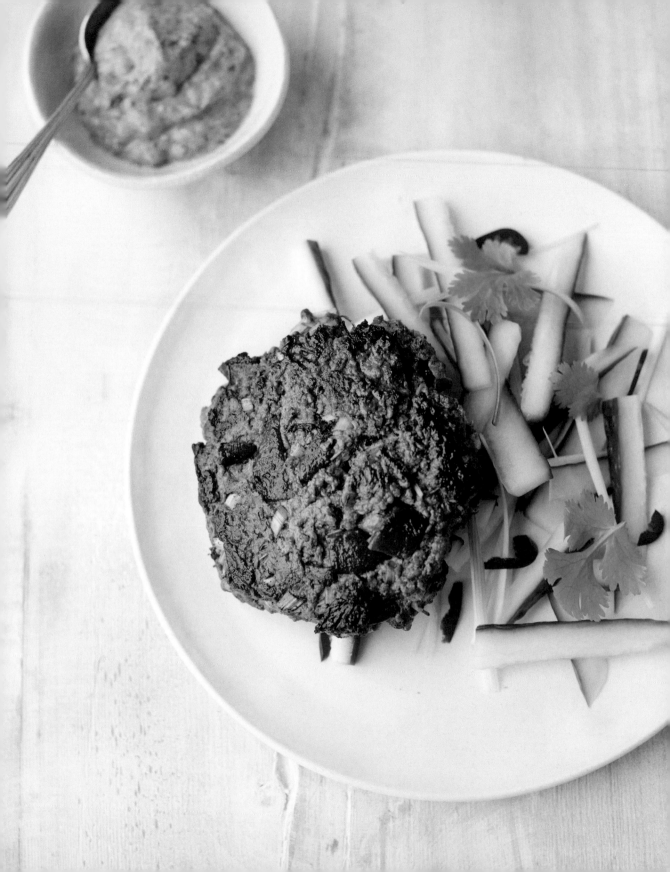

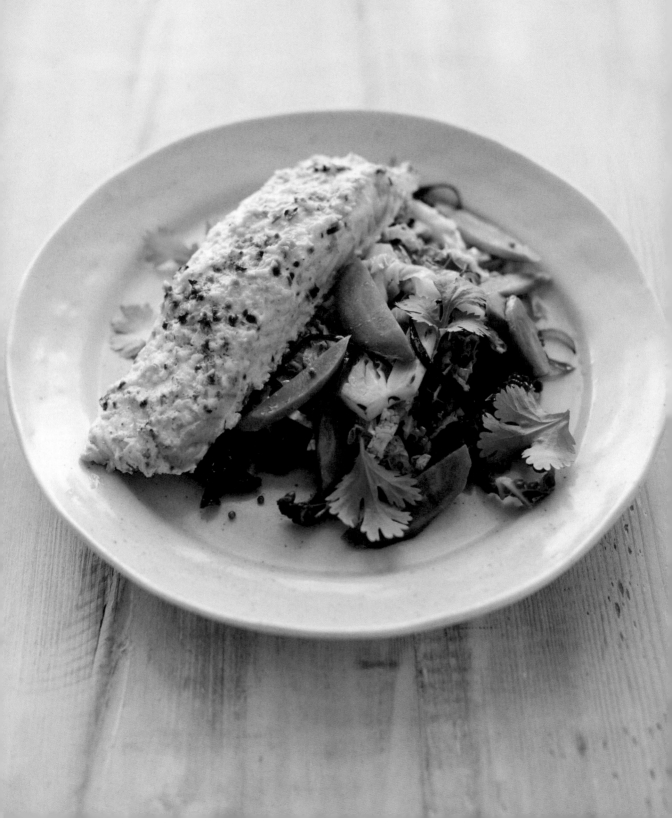

TANDOORI FISH
WITH QUICK VEG THORAN

SERVES

2

For the fish
2 x 130g boneless salmon
   fillets, cod loin or other
   firm fish, skin left on
1 lime, juice only
pinch of flaked sea salt,
   such as Maldon
1 mild green chilli, seeds
   removed, roughly
   chopped
4cm piece ginger, peeled
   and roughly chopped
½ small red onion,
   roughly chopped

1 clove garlic, roughly
   chopped
1 teaspoon garam masala
5 tablespoons unsweetened
   natural yoghurt (about
   4% fat)

For the thoran
100% mild and light olive
   oil spray
½ teaspoon mustard seeds
½ small red onion,
   thinly sliced

200g savoy cabbage, core
   removed, thinly shredded
2 medium carrots, halved
   lengthways then thinly
   sliced at an angle
1 teaspoon garam masala
pinch of flaked sea salt,
   such as Maldon

To serve
small handful fresh
   coriander, tender stalks
   and leaves
½ lime, cut into wedges

Thoran just means a 'dry' vegetable curry. This is an easy way to get loads of extra veggies into a meal. You can use any firm-fleshed fish for this dish – I love salmon or cod but look out for haddock, hake or pollack too. Try and buy sustainable fish if you can – ask at the fish counter or check the labelling.

* * *

1 Preheat a fan oven to 220°C or a grill to medium-high.

2 Place the fish on a non-stick roasting tray, squeeze the lime juice over the fish, then sprinkle with a pinch of salt. Set aside to marinate while you prepare the paste.

3 Tip the remaining fish ingredients into a mini food processor and blitz to a thin paste.

4 Pour the paste over the fish and turn it to coat all sides.

CONTINUED OVERLEAF

5 Roast at the top of the oven for 12–14 minutes, or under the grill for 8–10 minutes, until the fish is tinged with brown and cooked through. To check, gently pull apart the thickest part of the fish; it should be firm and opaque but not dry.

6 While the fish is cooking, spray a large non-stick frying pan or wok lightly with oil and heat over a medium-high heat. Add the mustard seeds (careful they may spit) and fry for 30 seconds, then add the onion and fry for 2 minutes. Add the cabbage and carrots and cook over a high heat, stirring often, for 5 minutes until just cooked but still with some crunch. Stir through the garam masala, season with salt to taste, and remove from the heat.

7 Serve the tandoori fish alongside the veg thoran and scatter with fresh coriander and lime wedges.

* * *

If you don't have a mini food processor make the paste by finely chopping the chilli and red onion and finely grating the ginger and garlic. Then just mix with the yoghurt.

* * *

WASABI SALMON AND PEAS
WITH ROASTED SWEET POTATO

SERVES

200g sweet potato, skin left
   on, cut into 2cm chunks
100% mild and light olive
   oil spray
2 x 130g boneless salmon
   fillets
pinch of flaked sea salt,
   such as Maldon

freshly ground black pepper
½ teaspoon paprika
   (optional)
1 tablespoon wasabi paste,
   made from powder
4 tablespoons
   unsweetened natural
   yoghurt (about 4% fat)

3 tablespoons chopped
   dill fronds
200g frozen peas
large handful pea shoots
   or watercress, reserve
   a few stalks to garnish

**The heat of the wasabi is matched
wonderfully here with the sweetness
of the sweet potato and peas. Pea
shoots are packed with vitamins A and
C and have a great flavour. They have
had a surge in popularity recently and
are available in many supermarkets.
However if you can't get hold of them
watercress will work just as well.**

* * *

1 Preheat a fan oven to 200°C.

2 Place the sweet potato into a non-
stick oven dish and spray to coat with
oil. Cook in the oven for 25 minutes.

3 Using your hands, coat each salmon
fillet with a few sprays of oil and place
skin side down into a non-stick oven dish
then season with salt and pepper. If
using the paprika gently pat it on top of
each fillet. Once the potatoes have been
cooking for 15 minutes add the salmon
to the oven for the remaining 10 minutes.

4 Meanwhile mix the wasabi paste
with the yoghurt and dill and set aside.

5 Half fill a medium pan with water
and bring to the boil. Add the peas
and return to the boil for 3 minutes.

6 Reserving a small cup of cooking
water; drain the peas and place them
back into the hot pan without heat. Add
the wasabi yoghurt and pea shoots into
the peas and stir to combine. Cover
with a lid.

7 Peel the skin from the salmon and,
using two forks, break gently into large
flakes. Add to the pan with the peas,
stir to combine adding a little of the
reserved cooking water to loosen
if necessary.

8 Arrange the sweet potatoes onto
warmed plates followed by the salmon
and peas. Garnish with extra pea shoots.

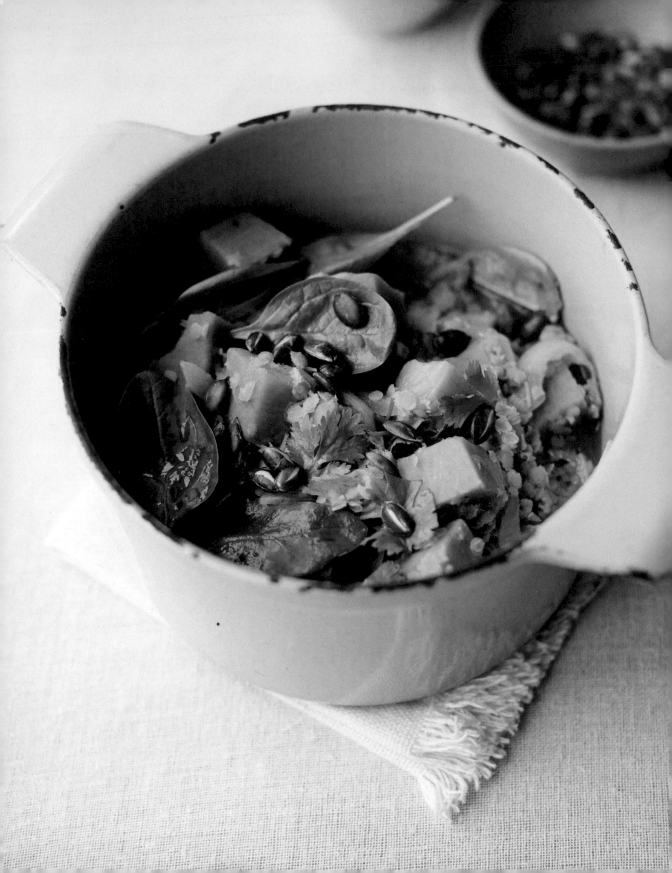

LENTIL AND SWEET POTATO STEW

10g pumpkin seeds
2 teaspoons mild olive oil
1 medium onion, sliced
1 clove garlic, finely chopped
1 teaspoon sweet smoked
    paprika or ½ teaspoon
    chipotle chilli powder
150g dried split red lentils,
    rinsed in water

300g sweet potato,
    skin left on, cut into
    2cm chunks
2 teaspoons vegetable
    bouillon powder
pinch of flaked sea salt,
    such as Maldon
freshly ground black pepper
100g baby spinach

large handful fresh
    coriander, tender stalks
    and leaves chopped, plus
    a few leaves to garnish
2 tablespoons unsweetened
    natural yoghurt (about
    4% fat) (optional)
1 lime, cut into wedges

**This one-pot stew is so easy to make
and really satisfying – perfect healthy
comfort food. The split red lentils don't
need soaking and cook in the stew in
about 15 minutes.**

* * *

1 To toast the seeds heat a fan oven
to 180°C, spread them on a baking tray
and toast for 5–7 minutes, stirring once,
or until lightly toasted. Or you can toss
them in a non-stick frying pan over a
medium heat for 5 minutes. Set aside.

2 Heat the olive oil in a large non-stick
saucepan or flameproof casserole over
a medium heat. Add the onions and
garlic and fry for 7–8 minutes. Be sure
to cook your onions until they're golden-
brown, it adds loads of extra flavour.

3 Stir in the smoked paprika and fry for
30 seconds then add the red lentils and
sweet potato and stir for a minute.

4 Pour in 700ml boiling water, stir in
the bouillon and increase the heat to
high. Once the stew is bubbling give it a
stir then reduce the heat to low-medium.
Cover the pan and cook for 20 minutes,
stirring every now and then. You might
need to add a splash more boiling water;
you're aiming for a nice, thick stew but
still with a bit of liquid.

5 Check the lentils and potato are tender
and season to taste. Stir in the spinach,
turn off the heat and leave to rest for
a minute.

6 Spoon into bowls and scatter over the
pumpkin seeds and coriander. Top with
a tablespoon of yoghurt if you like and
serve with the lime wedges on the side.

* * *

*You can toast a whole bag of pumpkin
seeds at a time and keep for up to three weeks
in an airtight container.*

* * *

VEGGIE PILAF
WITH CARAMELIZED ONIONS

2 teaspoons mild olive oil or vegetable oil

1 medium onion, thinly sliced

2 teaspoons ground cumin

1 teaspoon ground turmeric

½ teaspoon ground cloves

5cm piece cinnamon stick

3 cardamom pods, lightly crushed with the back of a spoon (optional)

2 medium carrots, cut into 1cm chunks

30g dried cherries, dried cranberries or dried blueberries

120g brown basmati rice

1 heaped teaspoon vegetable bouillon powder

200g cauliflower, broken into small florets

100g frozen peas, defrosted

about 15 fresh mint leaves

10g pistachio nut kernels, chopped

This is a fantastic vegetarian dish and proof they don't have to be boring. The sour dried cherries complement the spices perfectly.

* * *

1 Heat the oil in a large non-stick saucepan or flameproof casserole over a medium-high heat. Add the onions and fry for 10 minutes, stirring occasionally, until softened and golden-brown (don't rush this stage). Remove about half the onions and set aside.

2 Add all the spices to the pan containing the remaining onions and fry for 1 minute (if it looks like they might burn add a tablespoon or two of water).

3 Add the carrots, cherries and rice and stir around for a minute then pour in 425ml boiling water and the bouillon powder. Bring to the boil then turn the heat to medium. Stir, cover with a lid and simmer quite vigorously for 20 minutes.

4 After 20 minutes scatter the cauliflower florets over the top of the rice, put the lid back on and cook for a further 10 minutes. By now the rice should be just tender and most of the water absorbed; if it needs longer then add a splash more boiling water and cook for 5 more minutes. Finally, add the peas, cover and cook for 3 minutes.

4 Use a fork to gently fold the cauliflower and peas into the rice with half the mint. Scatter over the remaining mint, pistachios and the reserved caramelized onions.

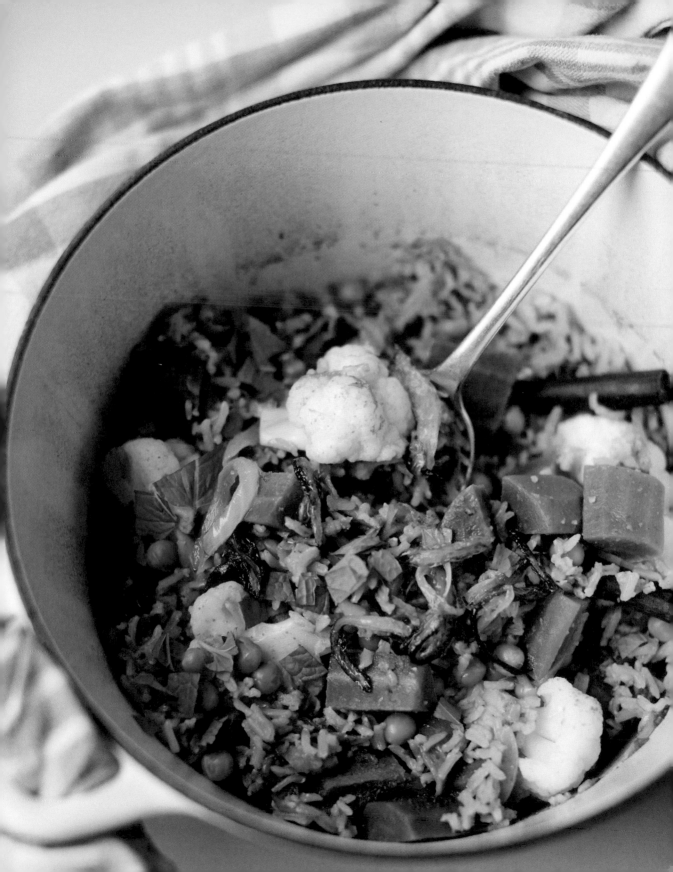

HONEY AND WHOLEGRAIN MUSTARD ROAST SALMON
WITH LEMON AND DILL BASHED POTATOES

SERVES

2

For the potatoes
400g new potatoes, skins left on, cut into 2cm chunks
pinch of flaked sea salt, such as Maldon
1 lemon, finely grated zest and juice
1 teaspoon chopped dill fronds

100% extra virgin olive oil spray
freshly ground black pepper

For the salmon
1 tablespoon wholegrain mustard
1 tablespoon freshly squeezed lemon juice

1 teaspoon runny honey
1 teaspoon mild or extra virgin olive oil
2 x 130g boneless salmon fillets, skin left on
pinch of flaked sea salt, such as Maldon
freshly ground black pepper

This Scandi-inspired recipe is one of my favourite dinners. It's so good you'd never know you were on a diet! Choose the thick-cut fillets of salmon rather than the thinner tail-end pieces if you can, although both will taste great. If using the tail-end pieces then reduce the cooking time by about 3 minutes. I always have it with whatever green vegetables are in season – tenderstem broccoli or green beans both work well.

★ ★ ★

1 Preheat a fan oven to 200°C.

2 Put the potatoes into a saucepan, cover with boiling water and season with salt. Bring to the boil and cook for 10 minutes until tender. Drain really thoroughly and return to the pan.

3 Stir through the lemon zest and juice, half the dill and plenty of freshly ground black pepper. Tip onto a large non-stick roasting tin then use a potato masher or the back of a fork to break the potatoes up a bit. Spray with oil. Roast in the oven for 12 minutes.

4 While the potatoes are roasting mix together the mustard, lemon juice, honey and oil. Place the salmon, skin-side down, on a non-stick roasting tin. Season with a little salt and pepper then spoon over the mustard mixture.

5 Once the potatoes have been cooking for 12 minutes, stir them around on the tray. Return them to the oven along with the salmon and cook both for 12 minutes.

6 To serve, sprinkle the remaining dill over the potatoes and serve alongside the salmon.

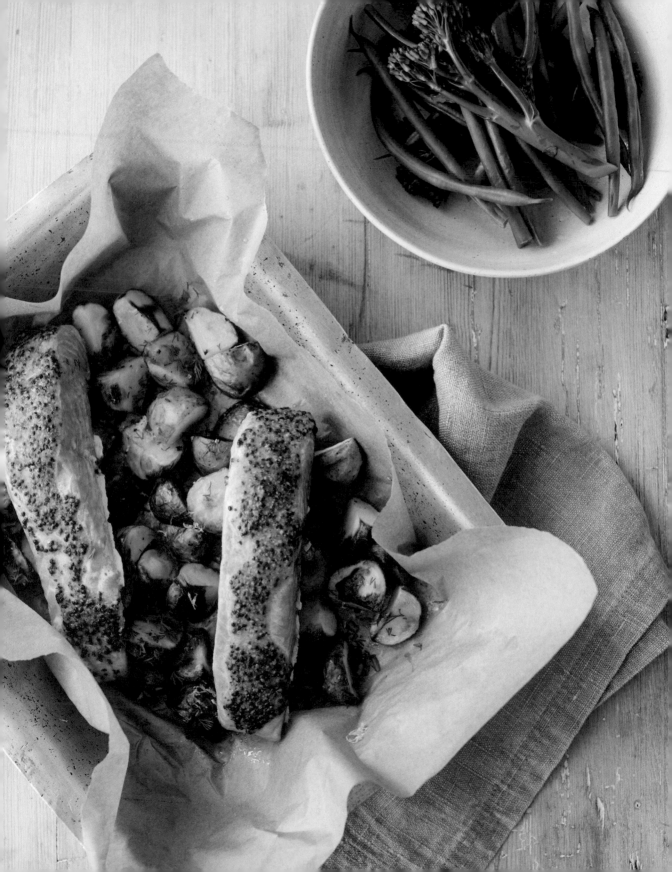

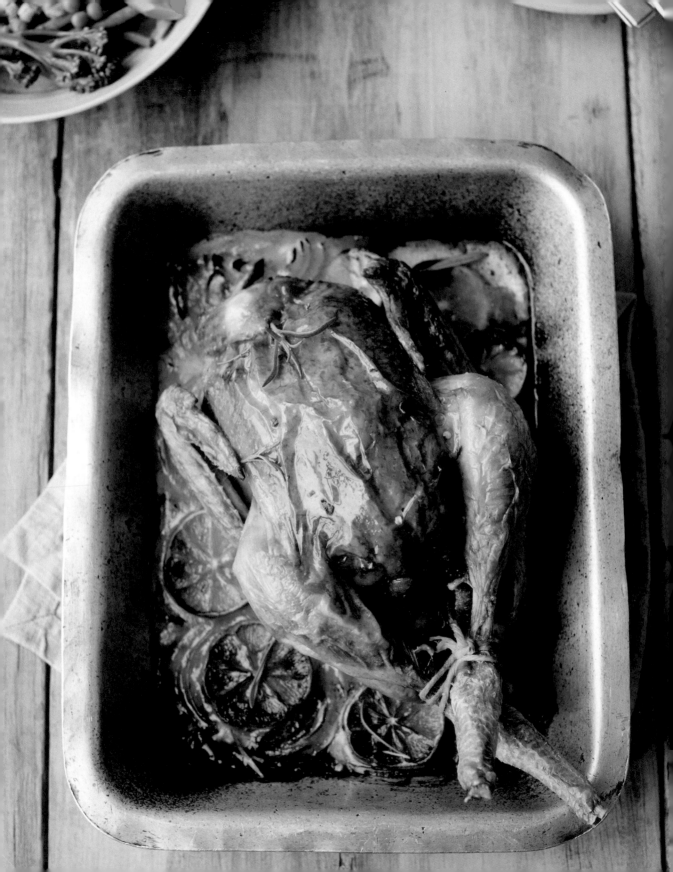

WHOLE ROAST CHICKEN
WITH HOT GREEN SALAD

SERVES

4

For the chicken
1 large onion, thinly sliced
2 lemons, juice of one
    and the other sliced
few sprigs fresh rosemary
    and/or thyme
100% mild and light olive
    oil spray
1 small free-range chicken
    (approx. 1.2 kg)

pinch of flaked sea salt,
    such as Maldon
freshly ground black pepper
1 teaspoon dried chilli flakes

For the salad
150g green beans, trimmed
150g tenderstem broccoli
    and/or asparagus,
    trimmed
100g frozen peas

For the dressing
1 shallot, finely chopped
    (optional)
1 tablespoon balsamic
    vinegar
1 small orange, finely grated
    zest and 2 tablespoons
    juice
pinch of flaked sea salt,
    such as Maldon
freshly ground black pepper

Who doesn't love the smell of a roast dinner cooking in the oven? I love cooking it this way with onions, lots of lemon and a sprinkling of chilli flakes, taking it to a whole new level. This can be shared with friends or cooked for the family; just make sure you stick with the breast meat – remove the skin and trim off any fat – and you can still enjoy this treat.

★ ★ ★

1 Preheat a fan oven to 200°C.

2 Scatter the onions, lemon slices and whole stalks of rosemary and/or thyme over the base of a small roasting tin. Lightly spray with the olive oil and toss to coat. Place the chicken on top, breast-side-down. Pour the lemon juice over the chicken and onions etc. and season with salt and freshly ground black pepper. Roast in the oven for 30 minutes, checking after 15 minutes that there is enough liquid in the tin to stop the pan juices burning and adding a splash of boiling water if needed.

CONTINUED OVERLEAF

3 Turn the chicken breast-side-up, giving the onions etc. a stir. Spoon the juices over the chicken, season the breasts with salt and freshly ground black pepper and sprinkle with the chilli flakes. Return the chicken to the oven for 20 minutes or until the skin is crisp and golden and the chicken is completely cooked through (the legs should pull away easily from the carcass and there should be no bloody juices). Take the chicken out of the oven and leave it to rest.

4 While the chicken is resting bring a large pan of salted water to the boil, add the green beans and broccoli or asparagus and boil for 3 minutes then add the peas and cook for a further minute. The veg should be just tender but still with some crunch.

5 To make the dressing, whisk together all the ingredients, or tip into a jam jar, screw the lid on tightly and shake well.

6 Drain the vegetables thoroughly, return to the pan and toss through the dressing.

7 Carve the chicken. Spoon any excess oil from the roasting tin then pour the remaining juices over the chicken.

8 Transfer to serving bowls and serve with the hot green salad.

* * *

Be sure to rest the chicken for 5–10 minutes before you carve it; this allows the chicken to become extra tender and the juices to collect in the roasting tin.

* * *

KING PRAWN AND NOODLE STIR FRY

SERVES

2

40g dried instant vermicelli rice noodles

230g raw king prawns, defrosted if frozen, blotted dry with kitchen paper

1½ tablespoons tamarind paste, or equivalent in freshly squeezed lime juice

freshly ground black pepper

100% mild and light olive oil spray

½ teaspoon turmeric

1 teaspoon hot curry powder

1 teaspoon dried chilli flakes

2cm piece ginger, peeled and cut into fine matchsticks

2 cloves garlic, finely chopped

½ small red onion, sliced

1 medium carrot, cut into matchsticks and blotted dry with kitchen paper

50g frozen peas

1 small courgette, grated and placed between kitchen paper to extract moisture

1 medium free-range egg, lightly beaten

1 teaspoon toasted sesame oil

This is reminiscent of Singapore noodles – skinny style! There doesn't need to be loads of oil for a dish like this to taste sensational. Tamarind, used here, is popular across the world and widely available in many supermarkets as a runny paste in a jar. It has a sweet yet predominantly sour taste, if you can't find it use the equivalent quantity of fresh lime juice instead.

★ ★ ★

1 Cover the instant noodles in boiling water for 2 minutes then drain and plunge into cold water. Drain well and spread out across kitchen paper to dry.

2 Place the prawns in a medium bowl and coat with 1 tablespoon of the tamarind paste, a few twists of black pepper and a few sprays of oil. Set aside.

3 Combine the turmeric, hot curry powder and chilli flakes in a bowl. Set aside.

4 Place a large non-stick frying pan or wok over a medium-high heat and spritz with oil. Add the ginger and garlic for 30 seconds followed by the onion, carrot and spices. Stir fry for another 30 seconds.

CONTINUED OVERLEAF

5 If required add a little more oil, then the prawns; cook for another minute. Follow with the noodles, peas and courgette and mix well over the heat for 30 seconds. Keep everything moving so it cooks evenly – a pair of kitchen tongs will help get the noodles incorporated with everything else.

6 Make a space at the bottom of the pan and pour in the egg, cook for 30 seconds and then use one chopstick to scramble it. Stir the egg into the noodles and veg. Now add the remaining tamarind paste and sesame oil and mix through.

7 Serve in heated bowls and eat with chopsticks!

* * *

Have everything ready and next to the hob before you start cooking, including the oil in case you need a few extra sprays.

* * *

LAMB TAGINE
WITH POTATOES AND PEAS

SERVES

500ml vegetable stock
(choose very good quality
organic stock cubes)
30g dried prunes, pitted
and halved
100% mild and light olive
oil spray

1 red onion, sliced into rings
¼ teaspoon ground
cinnamon
½ teaspoon whole cumin
seeds
250g lamb leg steak, fat
trimmed and diced

200g small waxy potatoes
(e.g. Charlotte), skins
left on, quartered
1 aubergine, cut into
2cm chunks
handful frozen peas
about 10 fresh mint leaves

Native to Morocco, a tagine is a slow cooked stew that takes its name from the conical shaped dish that is traditionally used. However, you don't need hours or special equipment to cook one. A wide shallow cast-iron casserole pan with a tight-fitting lid is perfect and it can be on the table in an hour. As everything is cooked in one pot, not only is it easy, but all of the nutrients are kept. It's all you need for a beautifully spiced delicate stew that can be enjoyed by all the family.

* * *

1 Pour the stock over the prunes so they can plump up. Set aside.

2 Using a wide shallow cast-iron pan that has a tight-fitting lid add the olive oil and set over a medium heat. Add the onions; when starting to soften and pick up some colour add the cinnamon and cumin and mix gently.

3 Turn the heat to low and add the lamb and gently colour, there is no need to season the meat at this point as the stock will be salty enough. Once the lamb has browned pour over the stock and prunes, and mix. Tuck the potatoes into the thin gravy and scatter the aubergine over the top to steam. Cover with the tight-fitting lid. Increase the heat a little and simmer for about 30 minutes. Check a few times and add just-boiled water if more liquid is needed.

4 After 30 minutes scatter the frozen peas into the pan, cover and switch off the heat. Leave for about 3 minutes.

5 Sprinkle the tagine with mint leaves and serve in warm bowls.

SPEEDY THAI-STYLE SALMON
WITH GREEN VEG STIR FRY

SERVES

2

For the marinade
large handful fresh
   coriander, tender stalks
   and leaves finely chopped
½ mild red chilli, seeds
   removed, finely chopped
4cm piece ginger, peeled
   and finely grated
1 clove garlic, finely chopped
1 tablespoon dark soy sauce

For the stir fry
100% mild and light olive
   oil spray
2 spring onions, outer
   leaves and tops removed,
   green and white parts
   finely chopped
250g mixed green
   vegetables
about 15 fresh mint leaves

1 tablespoon freshly
   squeezed lime juice
1 teaspoon toasted sesame
   oil (optional)
½ mild red chilli, seeds
   removed, thinly sliced

To finish
2 x 130g boneless salmon
   fillets, skin removed

**This is just the dish to have up your
sleeve for after work. Choose nice chunky
salmon fillets, not the thin tail-end
pieces. You can use a mixture of green
vegetables depending on what you
have to hand. Mangetout or sugar snaps
work well as do small broccoli florets
or defrosted frozen peas.**

* * *

1 Mix all the marinade ingredients
together and set aside.

2 Spray a non-stick frying pan or wok
lightly with oil and set over a high heat.
Add the spring onions and vegetables
and fry, stirring often, for 5 minutes.
They should be just cooked through but
still with crunch. Tear in the mint leaves,
squeeze over the lime juice and toss
with the toasted sesame oil if using.

3 Divide the stir fry between two serving
plates and scatter with the red chilli.

4 Cut each salmon fillet in half
lengthways so you have four evenly
sized long, thin 'fingers' of salmon.
Meanwhile, bring a large pan of water
to a simmer. Add the salmon and cook
for exactly one minute, or two minutes
if you like it firm all the way through.
Remove with a slotted spoon and
arrange two pieces on each plate.

5 Spoon the marinade over the
salmon and serve.

* * *

*Use a mini food processor to make the marinade
to save time. Just roughly chop the ingredients
and blitz to a coarse paste, adding a splash
of cold water to loosen if needed.*

* * *

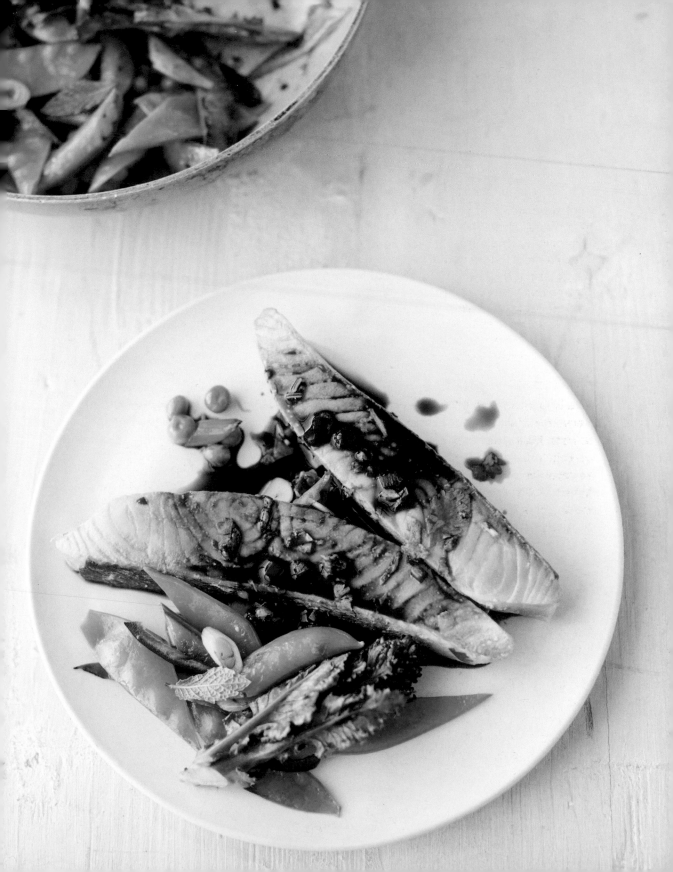

SPICY HARISSA PRAWNS
WITH LEMON QUINOA

For the quinoa
80g quinoa, rinsed under
    cold water
100g frozen peas, defrosted
2 tablespoons freshly
    squeezed lemon juice
small handful soft green
    herbs, roughly chopped,
    plus a few extra to garnish

pinch of flaked sea salt,
    such as Maldon

For the prawns
100% mild and light olive
    oil spray
1 red romero pepper,
    seeds removed,
    thinly sliced

200g raw peeled king
    prawns, frozen or
    defrosted
1 tablespoon red or rose
    harissa paste

This spicy dish is so quick and packed with flavour. All harissas vary in their spiciness so the amount you'll need will depend on the brand. Start off with a tablespoon and add more if it's not too spicy. I use whatever herbs I've got in my fridge, or can grab easily at the shops. Try coriander, dill, flatleaf parsley or mint, or a mixture of them all! You could swap the quinoa for the same quantity of wholewheat couscous prepared according to packet instructions.

★ ★ ★

1 Tip the quinoa into a pan with 240ml cold water (or according to packet instructions). Bring to the boil then lower to a simmer, cover the pan and cook for 15 minutes or until most of the water has been absorbed. Add the peas, cover and cook for a further 2 minutes then stir in the lemon juice, chopped herbs and salt, to taste. Set aside.

2 For the prawns, spray a non-stick frying pan lightly with the oil and place over a medium-high heat. When the pan is hot add the peppers and the prawns and fry for 1–2 minutes until just turning pink. Add the harissa paste and toss to coat thoroughly. Cook for a further minute or until the prawns are pink and opaque all the way through, adding a tablespoon or two of boiling water towards the end to prevent the harissa paste from burning. Let the water bubble, stir, then turn off the heat.

3 Serve the prawns on the quinoa and scattered with the remaining herbs.

★ ★ ★

You can use frozen, defrosted prawns for this recipe. Keep a bag in the freezer and a jar of harissa in your fridge and you'll always have something for dinner.

★ ★ ★

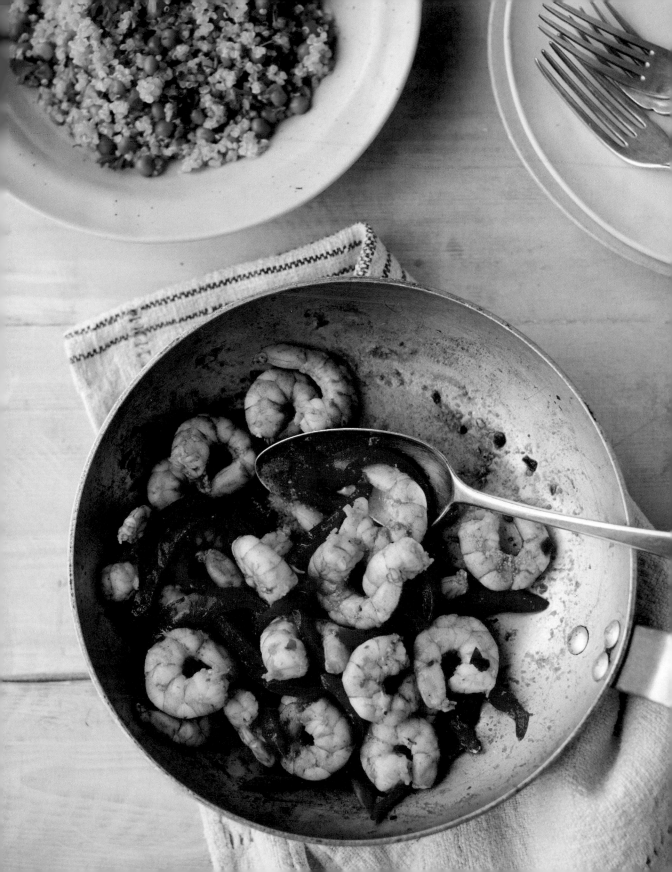

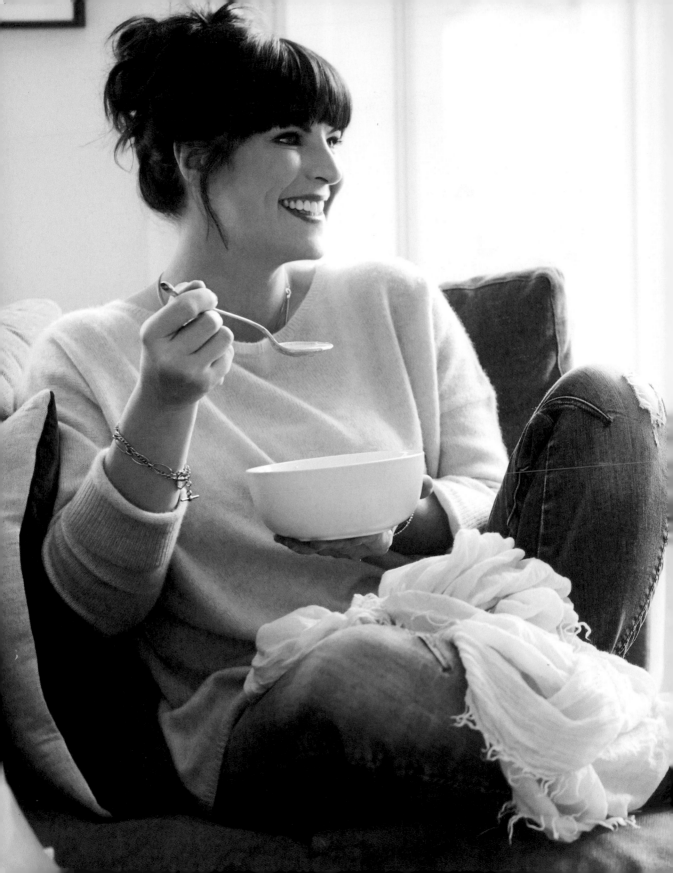

SOUPS

I've said it before, and I'll say it again: I have a bit of a thing about soups. More than a thing, it's a mild obsession. To my mind, they're a perfect meal in a bowl, and you can be so inventive about what to throw together.

I also love them because I find they tend to fill me up for longer, compared to a 'solid' meal of the same calorie equivalent.

The soups in this section, by the way, come in at under 300 calories per bowl. Use them as a light lunch, or supper option – that way you'll cut your overall daily calorie intake and drop the pounds that little bit faster. Or alternatively, a smaller portion can be eaten as a snack.

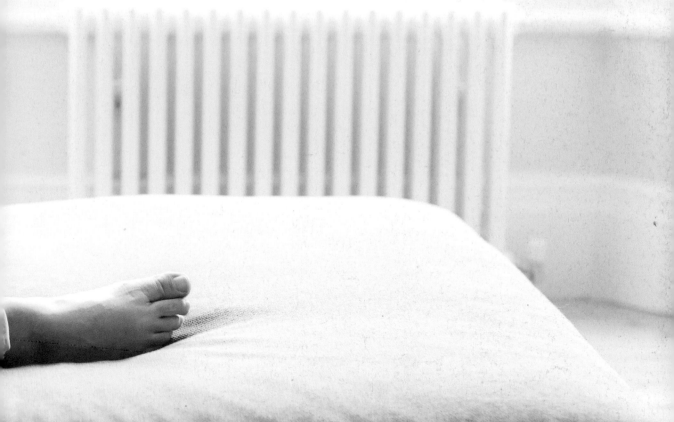

RED LENTIL AND COCONUT SOUP

SERVES

2

1 leek
2 teaspoons coconut oil
1 clove garlic, finely
    chopped
4cm piece ginger,
    peeled and grated
½ teaspoon turmeric

100g dried split red lentils,
    rinsed in water
100ml coconut milk
500ml vegetable stock
    (choose very good
    quality organic
    stock cubes)

For the garnish
1 teaspoon coconut oil
1 teaspoon mustard seeds
1 teaspoon dried chilli flakes
1 tablespoon fresh or dried
    curry leaves

Turmeric is renowned for its health benefits and healing properties. It shines in this warm comforting soup that will be enjoyed by all the family. Even babies and young children will be seduced by its sweet richness and gentle flavours. For older palettes add the tarka garnish to give it some heat!

* * *

1 Prepare the leek. Remove the top and, holding the root, cut into eight lengthways. Wash and finely slice.

2 Heat the coconut oil in a large non-stick saucepan or flameproof casserole over a medium heat and add the leek, garlic and ginger. After a couple of minutes turn to low and cook for 10 minutes until soft and translucent.

3 Stir in the turmeric, then add the lentils and stir again.

4 Mix in the coconut milk for a couple of minutes then add the stock and bring to the boil. Simmer gently uncovered for 10 minutes stirring occasionally or until the lentils are just under the surface.

5 For the garnish heat a small non-stick frying pan over a high heat, melt the teaspoon of coconut oil then add the mustard seeds, chilli flakes and curry leaves, cooking for a few minutes until fragrant.

6 Ladle into warmed bowls, and add the tarka to garnish.

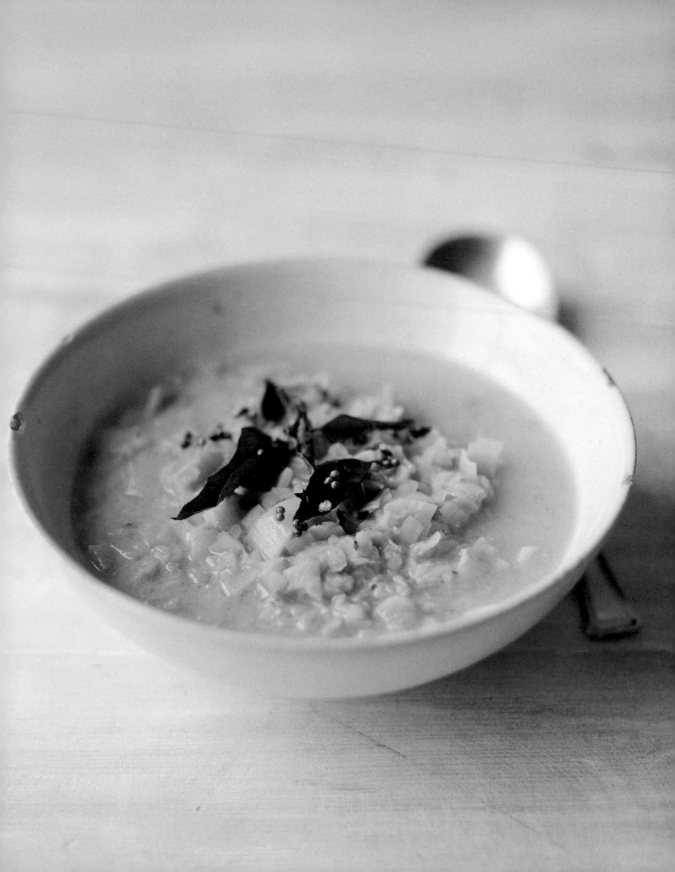

PEA AND WATERCRESS SOUP
WITH CRISPY PARMA HAM

SERVES

100% mild and light olive
   oil spray
1 small white onion,
   finely chopped
1 clove garlic, finely chopped

2 slices Parma ham
400ml chicken stock made
   from ½ a cube (choose
   very good quality organic
   stock cubes)

200g frozen petits pois
50g watercress, leaves and
   tender stalks, plus a few
   leaves to garnish

This bright green fresh pea soup has peppery warmth from the watercress and richness from the addition of Parma ham. Fresh enough to enjoy in the summer yet comforting during the winter months.

* * *

1 Lightly spray a medium non-stick frying pan with oil and, over a medium-low heat, gently sauté the onion and garlic for 5 minutes or until soft and translucent.

2 Transfer the onion mixture into a large saucepan and set aside.

3 Place the non-stick frying pan back onto a medium heat and add the Parma ham, cooking on each side for 3 minutes or until there is some colour. Set aside.

4 Meanwhile add the stock to the saucepan containing the onion mixture and bring to the boil. Once boiling add the peas and bring back to boiling again. Add the watercress and take off the heat.

5 Use a stick blender to blend to a smooth consistency.

6 Serve immediately in warmed bowls. Use scissors to snip the Parma ham into the centre of each bowl and garnish with the reserved watercress leaves.

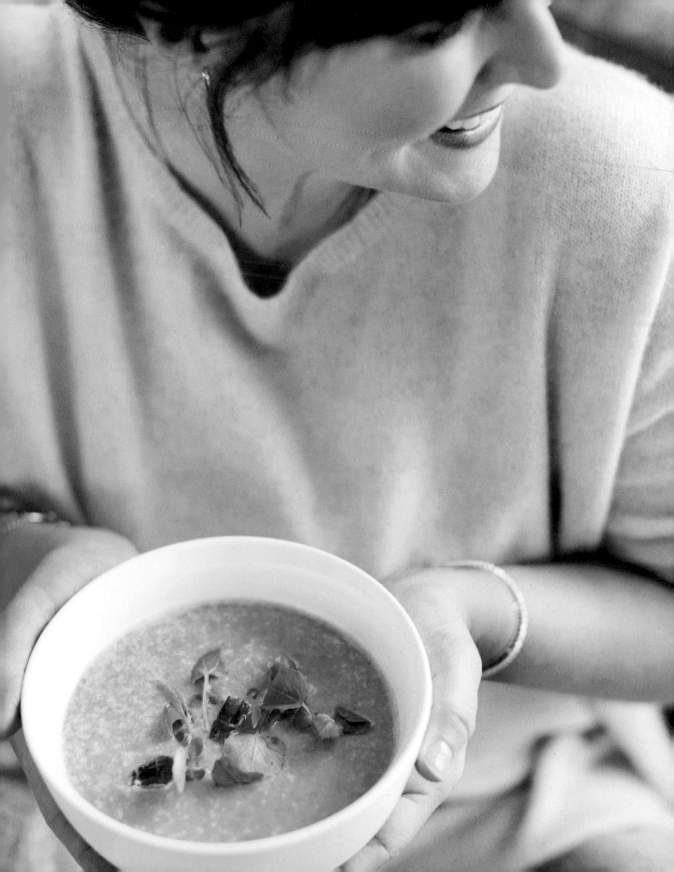

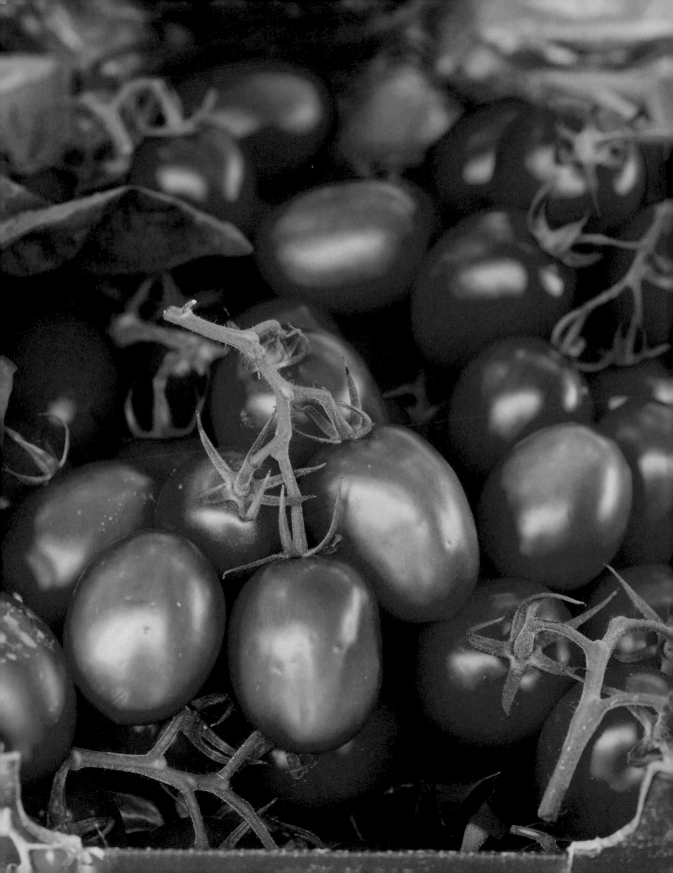

BEST-EVER ROAST TOMATO SOUP

SERVES

2

600g medium vine-
　ripened tomatoes,
　cut into quarters
150g peeled butternut
　squash or skin-on sweet
　potato, cut into 1cm
　cubes or thin slices

1 medium red onion,
　cut into 8 wedges
2 cloves garlic, skins left on
about 10 large basil leaves,
　plus 2 to serve
extra virgin olive oil
　spray

1 heaped teaspoon
　vegetable bouillon
　powder
pinch of flaked sea salt,
　such as Maldon
freshly ground black
　pepper

Roasting the tomatoes makes this soup really tasty. Try and choose tomatoes with plenty of flavour. Vine-ripened tomatoes are a pretty good bet, otherwise be sure they have a nice deep red colour and a lovely fragrance to them. I like to add some butternut squash or sweet potato to give it a really thick consistency and make it a bit more filling. They also balance the acidity of the tomatoes. You can buy ready peeled and chopped butternut squash in most supermarkets.

* * *

1 Preheat a fan oven to 200°C.

2 Toss all the ingredients, apart from the vegetable bouillon and seasoning, together in a large non-stick roasting tin. Roast in the oven for 20 minutes. Remove the garlic and set aside. Stir everything else and return to the oven for a further 10–15 minutes, until everything is just tinged golden-brown and the tomatoes collapsed and sticky.

3 Scrape the contents of the roasting tin into a large saucepan. Mash some of the tomatoes in the tin so they release some juice and use this to help lift off any sticky bits on the bottom of the pan – they'll be full of flavour! Add 500–600ml boiling water and the vegetable bouillon to the pan. Squeeze the garlic cloves out of their papery skins and add these too.

4 Simmer the contents of the pan over a medium heat for 5 minutes then turn off the heat and blend to a smooth consistency using a stick blender. Taste for seasoning and add some salt if needed. Add plenty of freshly ground black pepper.

5 Ladle into warm bowls, top each with a basil leaf and serve.

GREEN MINESTRONE

SERVES

2

1 teaspoon olive oil
4 spring onions, outer
    leaves and tops removed,
    green and white parts
    finely sliced
1 courgette, cut into
    1cm chunks
100g green beans, trimmed
    and cut into 2cm pieces

100g frozen peas
50g dark greens (e.g. savoy
    cabbage, spring greens,
    cavolo nero), thinly
    shredded
1 x 400g tin white beans
    such as cannellini
    or haricot, drained
    and rinsed

2 teaspoons vegetable
    bouillon powder
pinch of flaked sea salt,
    such as Maldon
freshly ground black pepper
about 10 basil leaves

**This soup is packed full of veggies and
ready in 10 minutes – what's not to love!**

* * *

*For a lower calorie, but slightly less
filling option, you can leave out the white
beans and treat this as a snack.*

* * *

1 Heat the oil in a large non-stick saucepan
or flameproof casserole over a medium-
high heat. Add the spring onions and
courgette and fry for 4 minutes until
softened. Add all the remaining
vegetables, 450–550ml boiling water
and the bouillon powder. Bring to the
boil then lower the heat to medium and
boil gently for 5 minutes or until the
vegetables are just cooked through
but the beans still have a little crunch.

2 Taste the soup and add a little salt
if needed. Ladle into bowls, season
with freshly ground black pepper
and tear in the basil leaves.

SWEET POTATO SOUP
WITH TOASTED SEEDS

SERVES

10g pumpkin and/or
   sunflower seeds
100% mild and light olive
   oil spray
1 small red onion, quite
   finely chopped

350g sweet potatoes,
   skin left on, cut into
   2cm chunks
½ teaspoon mild chilli
   powder, paprika or sweet
   smoked paprika, plus a

pinch to serve
2 teaspoons vegetable
   bouillon powder
pinch of flaked sea salt,
   such as Maldon
freshly ground black pepper

**This soup is so quick and easy to make
and really filling. One of my fave lunches
on a cold day. You can jazz it up with
a squeeze of lime and some fresh
coriander if you like, and/or swap the
seeds for a tablespoon of natural plain
yoghurt swirled in just before serving.**

* * *

1 To toast the seeds either heat the
oven to 180°C, spread them on a baking
tray and toast them in the oven for 5–7
minutes, stirring once, or until lightly
toasted. Alternatively you can toss them
in a non-stick frying pan over a medium
heat for about 5 minutes until toasted.
Set aside.

2 For the soup, spray a little olive oil
in a non-stick saucepan or flameproof
casserole and place over a medium heat.
Add the onions and sweet potato and
fry for 2–3 minutes.

3 Stir in the chilli powder and bouillon
powder then pour in 550ml of boiling
water. Bring to the boil and simmer
for 15–20 minutes, or until the sweet
potato is completely tender.

4 Use a stick blender to blend to a
smooth consistency, adding a splash
more boiling water if you prefer a
thinner soup. Season with salt and
pepper, to taste.

5 Ladle into warm serving bowls and
sprinkle over the seeds and a small
pinch of chilli powder.

* * *

*If you're in a hurry for the soup you can coarsely
grate the sweet potato instead of chopping
it and cook until tender – about 10–12 minutes.*

* * *

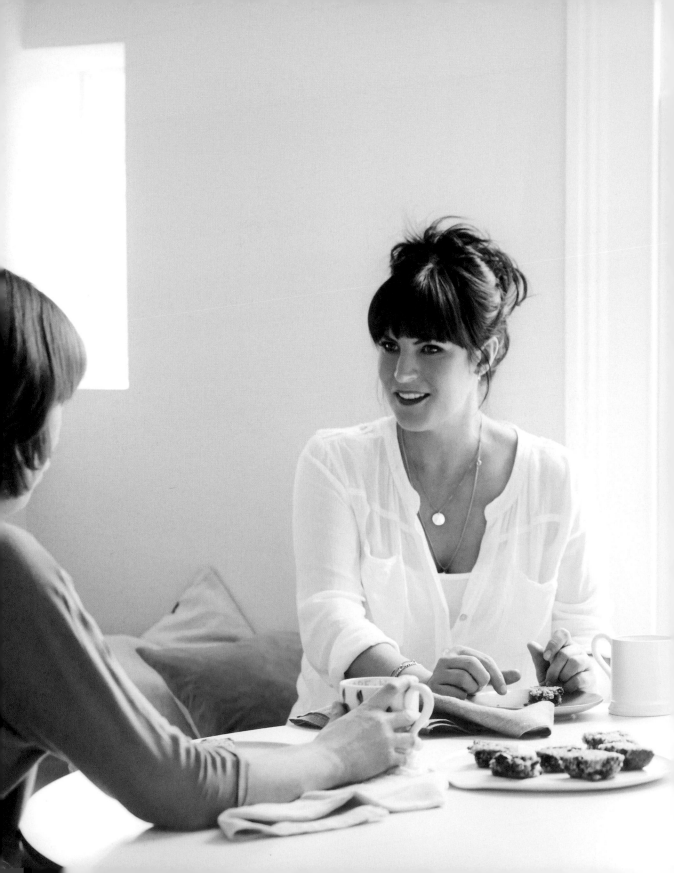

SNACKS

Mention the word 'snack' and most people think high-sugar, high-fat, high-carb indulgence – a cheeky treat to enjoy before the next proper meal comes along.

But my snacks are different. Cheeky, yes! But also healthy, nutritious and guilt-free. They're only 200 calories a pop, so enjoy one on top of your three meals a day. They may look sinful, but they'll keep your blood sugar – and your waistline – under control.

KALE CRISPS

100g kale (prepped weight), stalks removed, leaves torn
100% mild and light olive oil spray

generous pinch of flaked sea salt, such as Maldon
freshly ground black pepper
¼ teaspoon ground cumin

pinch garlic granules
pinch chilli powder

If you have a weakness for crisps, give these a try and see if they can replace that savoury taste that you crave. All of the nutrients remain in the kale and you can play around with the seasoning – try your favourite spice mix from Cajun to Ras el-hanout.

★ ★ ★

1 Preheat a fan oven and two baking trays to 200°C.

2 The kale needs to be washed and very thoroughly patted dry with a clean towel or simply left on a tray to air dry. Once the leaves are dry tip into a large bowl, spray the leaves with oil and massage in with your fingers. Season with salt and the spices and toss with your fingers to coat well.

3 Remove the two trays from the oven and line with baking paper and spread the kale out across the two trays.

4 Place the kale in the oven and immediately switch the oven off. Leave the kale leaves undisturbed in the oven for at least 1 hour, until they are crispy. They'll continue to crisp up afterwards too.

5 Serve in a bowl and share.

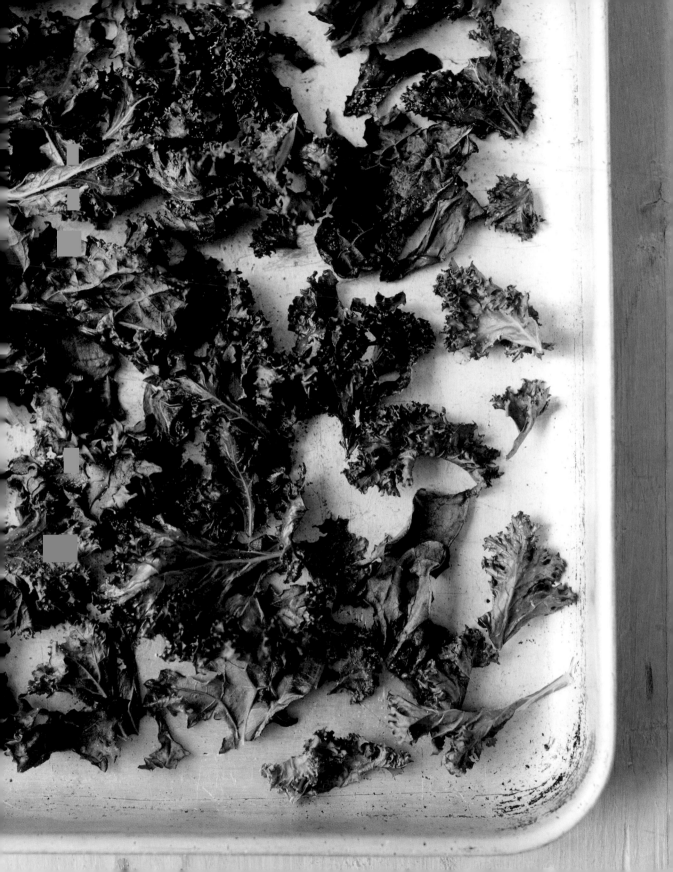

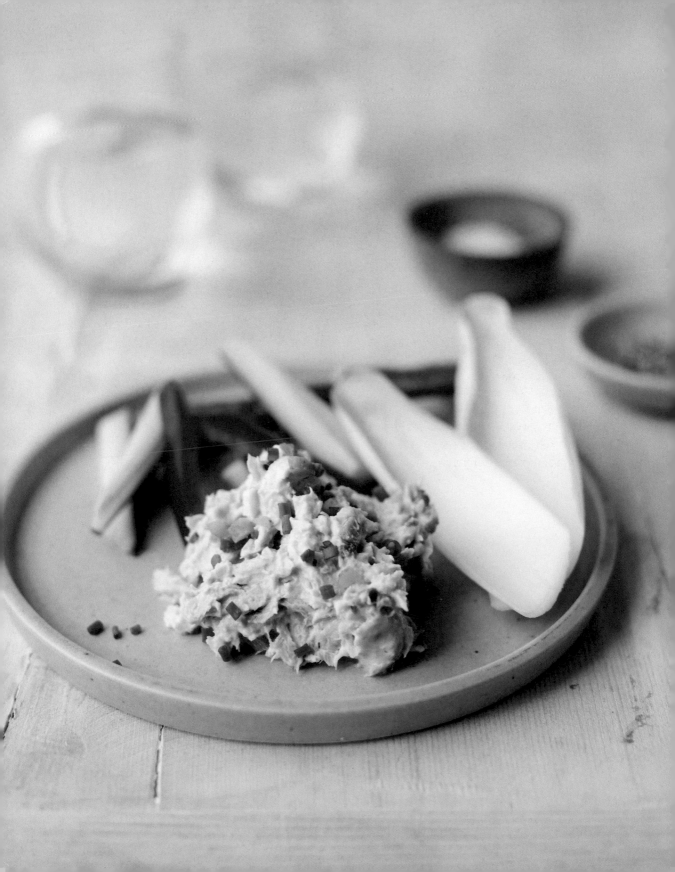

SMOKED FISH PÂTÉ

SERVES

2

75g hot smoked fish
fillets, skinless
2 tablespoons reduced-fat
cream cheese

1 tablespoon chives,
finely chopped
2 tablespoons pickled
gherkins, finely diced,
plus liquor

freshly ground black
pepper

This pâté can be made from hot smoked trout or salmon, but be aware that with salmon the calorie count will be higher than with trout, although still within the allowance. It makes a great snack with a selection of vegetables. Carrots or raw beetroot cut into batons work well, or try small, whole chicory leaves. For a more substantial lunch serve with crispbread and a green salad.

★ ★ ★

1 Flake the fish into a mixing bowl removing any obvious bones as you go, add the cream cheese and mix well with a fork.

2 Add the chives and gherkins and mix again, loosen with a couple of tablespoons of the gherkin liquor if necessary.

3 Season with freshly ground black pepper.

HOMEMADE HUMMUS

SERVES

4

2 tablespoons tahini
1 lemon, juice only
1 teaspoon salt

1 clove garlic, finely chopped
1 x 400g tin chickpeas,
    drained and water
    reserved

1 tablespoon mild
    olive oil

Hummus makes a nourishing wholesome snack to eat with vegetable crudités or use as part of a meal. It can also be varied with your favourite flavours. I've given you a couple of suggestions on the following page. It will keep well in the fridge for a few days.

* * *

1 In a small bowl mix the tahini with the lemon juice, half the salt and the garlic until thick. Loosen with about 4 tablespoons of the chickpea water from the can.

2 Combine this mixture with the chickpeas and using a stick blender or food processor blitz until smooth.

3 Stir in the tablespoon of olive oil and season with the remaining salt and lemon juice to taste.

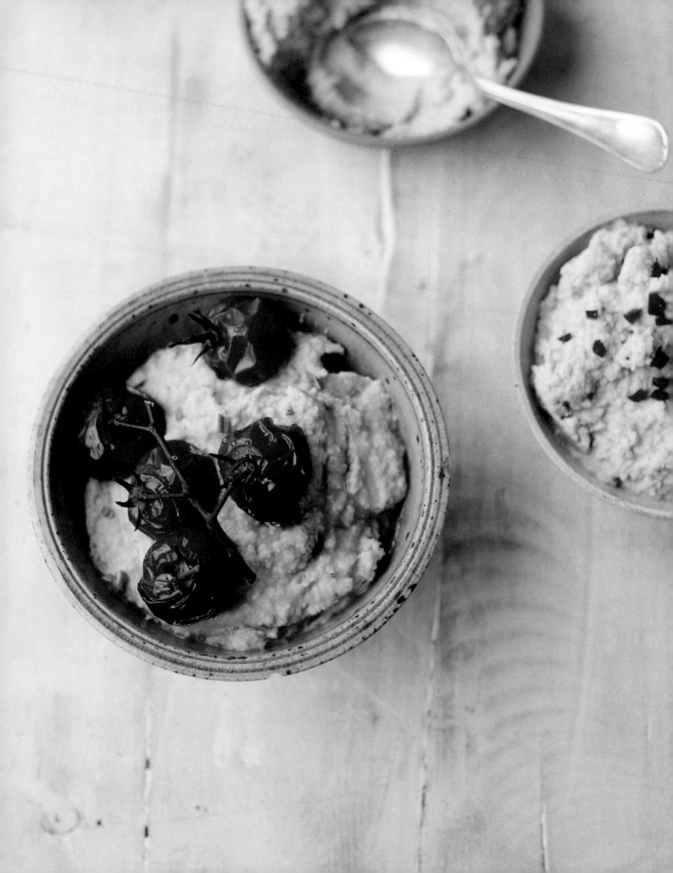

ROAST TOMATO
AND ROSEMARY HUMMUS

SERVES

150g small or medium
   vine-ripened tomatoes
100% mild and light olive
   oil spray

pinch of flaked sea salt,
   such as Maldon

1 heaped teaspoon
   fresh rosemary needles,
   finely chopped
1 batch Homemade hummus

This is a great way of incorporating a few tomatoes from your fridge drawer.

★ ★ ★

1 Preheat a fan oven to 200°C.

2 Place the tomatoes onto a baking sheet and spray with oil and season with salt. Roast for 20 minutes.

3 Reserve a small bunch of roasted tomatoes, then stir the remainder and the chopped rosemary into the basic hummus recipe before the final seasoning step. Top with with the reserved tomatoes.

SPICY HUMMUS

SERVES

4

1 red bird's eye chilli, seeds
   removed, finely chopped

1 teaspoon white wine
   vinegar

1 batch Homemade
   hummus

If you like things a little spicy, then this is the hummus for you.

★ ★ ★

1 Mix the chilli and vinegar together and stir into the basic hummus recipe before the final seasoning step.

ROAST AUBERGINE, LEMON AND GARLIC DIP

1 large aubergine, cut into
   2cm chunks
4 cloves garlic, skins left on
extra virgin olive oil spray
pinch of flaked sea salt,
   such as Maldon
1 spring onion, outer leaves
   and top removed, green
and white parts roughly
chopped, reserve a few
green slices to garnish
large handful flatleaf
   parsley, tender stalks
   and leaves chopped
1½ tablespoons freshly
   squeezed lemon juice
120g unsweetened natural
   yoghurt (about 4% fat)
½–1 mild red or green chilli,
   seeds removed, roughly
   chopped (optional)

This dip tastes gorgeously creamy. Serve with lots of raw veg crudités such as carrots, cucumber, cauliflower or peppers. You can add a small toasted wholemeal pitta bread or a crispbread as long as it doesn't exceed 85 calories. For variation you can add different herbs – try fresh mint leaves, dill or coriander or a mixture.

* * *

1 Preheat a fan oven to 200°C.

2 Spread the aubergines and garlic on a large non-stick roasting tin and spray with olive oil. Season with salt and toss together. Roast for 10 minutes until tinged golden then add 150ml water and cook for a further 10 minutes.

3 Allow to cool slightly, then tip into a food processor with all the remaining ingredients. Blitz everything together to a fairly smooth consistency, leaving a little bit of texture.

4 Serve garnished with the reserved spring onion slices.

ROAST CARROT AND CUMIN DIP

SERVES

2

400g carrots, cut into
   1cm rounds
4 cloves garlic, skins left on
1 teaspoon whole cumin
   seeds

pinch of flaked sea salt,
   such as Maldon
freshly ground black pepper
1 tablespoon extra virgin
   olive oil

3 tablespoons unsweetened
   natural yoghurt
   (about 4% fat)
1 tablespoon freshly
   squeezed lime juice

I vowed I'd never buy another shop-bought dip again after trying this recipe! It's packed with flavour and is uber good for you. You can easily double the quantities to make an extra batch. It keeps in the fridge for two or three days. You can vary it by stirring in some chopped herbs – coriander, parsley or mint would all work well. You could also swirl in a teaspoon of harissa paste for a spicier dip. Serve with sticks of cucumber, red pepper or raw cauliflower.

* * *

*Organic carrots always seem to have bags
more flavour than non-organic. As this dip is made
mostly of carrots, it's worth looking out for organic
and spending that little bit more if you can.*

* * *

1 Preheat a fan oven to 180°C.

2 Tip the carrots, garlic, cumin and the salt and pepper into a large non-stick roasting tin. Drizzle with the olive oil and toss really thoroughly to coat everything in the oil. Roast for 20 minutes until the garlic is tender. Remove the garlic and set aside to cool. Sprinkle 5 tablespoons of water over the carrots and roast for a further 10 minutes. Leave to cool slightly.

3 Tip the roasted carrots into a food processor. Squeeze the garlic cloves out of their papery skins and add to the carrots. Blend roughly then add the yoghurt, lime juice and 3–4 tablespoons of boiling water and blend until almost smooth but still with some texture. Taste for seasoning then transfer to a serving bowl.

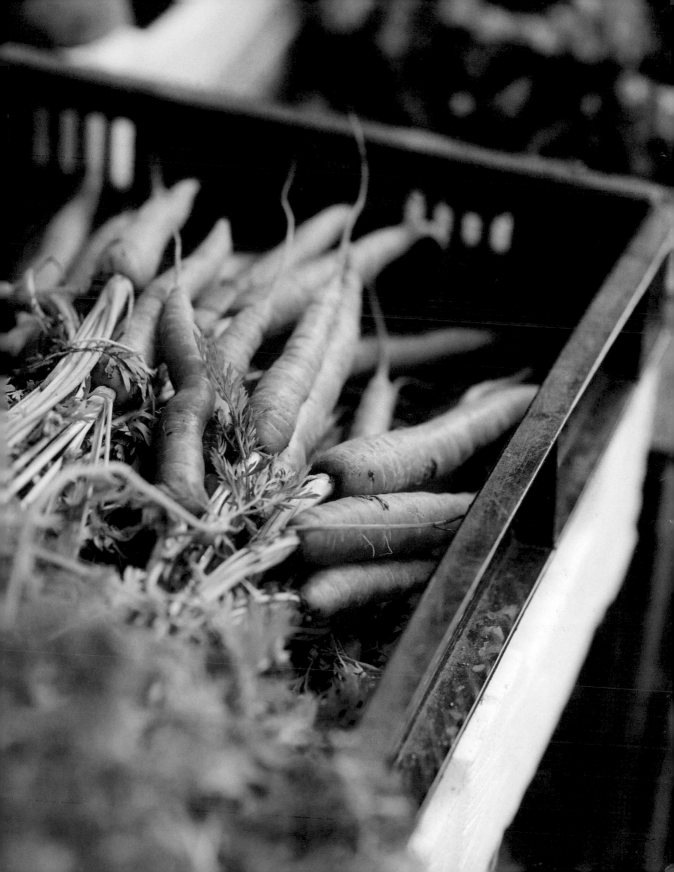

MINT TEA WITH DATE SQUARES

MAKES
16

For the date squares
100g pumpkin seeds

½ lime, finely grated zest,
if you like, and juice
200g dried pitted dates

For the tea
large handful fresh
mint leaves

If you have mint in the fridge or a forgotten mint plant in the garden then grab a good handful of leaves and infuse in boiling water, take a minute to yourself and enjoy the tea with one of these fudge size date squares, perfect when you need a little something sweet. Dates and pumpkin seeds are a wonderful combination; if you don't have time to make these squares a couple of dates and a few seeds will ward off hunger pains and are packed with nutrients.

* * *

These are great eaten straight from the freezer so make a batch and pop them in the freezer them for when you need a sweet treat!

* * *

1 Put the pumpkin seeds into a high-speed food processer and blitz until finely chopped, add in the lime juice and dates and process until the mixture forms a ball.

2 Drape some cling film over the edges of a small square foil tray or dish (approximately 12cm x 12cm) and press the mixture into the tray. Cover the mixture with the overhanging cling film and chill for at least 30 minutes, then cut into 16 squares. Return to the fridge, or freeze.

3 Place the mint leaves into cups or a teapot and pour over boiling water. Leave to infuse for a few minutes.

4 Enjoy the tea garnished with a few mint leaves and accompanied by a date square.

FIG, ORANGE AND PECAN FLAPJACKS

MAKES
12

1 large orange, finely
    grated zest and juice
2 tablespoons runny honey
50g dried figs, chopped
40g dried pitted dates,
    chopped

40g sultanas, chopped
2 tablespoons coconut oil
1 tablespoon sunflower oil
100g porridge oats (not
    jumbo)

15g chopped pecan nuts
few drops orange extract
    (optional)

**If you have a sweet tooth or just know
that you need a snack at certain points
in the day make a batch of these so that
you are not tempted with biscuits or
crisps; even one square with a cuppa
will take the edge off. They also double
as a good breakfast if you need to grab
something as you leave or prefer to eat
once you've been awake a few hours.**

* * *

1 Preheat a fan oven to 160°C. Line a
non-stick 900g loaf tin (approximately
22cm x 12cm x 7cm) with baking
parchment.

2 Put the orange zest and juice into a
small saucepan and add the honey, dried
fruit, coconut oil and sunflower oil. Heat
gently until bubbling – this takes about
4–5 minutes.

3 Put the oats, nuts and orange extract,
if using, into a bowl. Remove the pan
from the heat and pour the dried-fruit
mixture onto the oats mixture, mixing
well to combine.

4 Spoon the mixture into the loaf tin
and press down firmly. Bake for 30–35
minutes until golden.

5 Remove the tin from the oven and
set aside to cool. Once cool, remove
the flapjack from the loaf tin, holding
the sides of the parchment to lift it out.
Put on a board, and use a serrated bread
knife to cut it into six bars. Cut each bar
in half to make twelve squares. Store
in an airtight container, or freeze for
up to a month.

INDEX

addiction 39, 94
addictive eaters 28, 29, 34–5
alcohol 58, 84–5, 94, 95
appetite 82–3, 84–5
apples: apple and lime salsa 166
  dairy-free date and apple
    porridge 109
  simple green smoothie 121
Asian beef burger 172
Atkins Diet 27
aubergines: hot roast
    vegetable curry 167–8
  roast aubergine, lemon and
    garlic dip 213
  roasted vegetable and Puy
    lentil salad 128
Auditory Digital
  Representational System
  50, 52
Auditory Representational
  System 50, 51
avocado and bacon on rye
  toast 106

bacon: avocado and bacon on
  rye toast 106
bananas: ricotta, bananas and
  honey on rye toast 117
beach body countdown 21
beef: lean Asian beef burger 172
  toasted cashew and red chilli
    beef 136
  my favourite ragu with spelt
    pasta 162
beetroot: Scandi beetroot and
  smoked salmon mini
  frittata 154
berry and vanilla smoothie 122
Bircher muesli, blueberry and
  pistachio 118

black beans: Mexican street
    food tacos 148
  ultimate veggie burger
    169–70
blood sugar levels 27, 80, 85, 86
blueberry and pistachio
  Bircher 118
body language 58
brain: cravings 39
  neurotransmitters 34
  processing information 50
  recognizing 'fullness' 82–3
  tiredness 86–7
  see also subconscious mind
breakfast sundae 115
broccoli: hot green bean and
  feta salad 135
  hot green salad 185–6
burgers: lean Asian beef
  burger 172
  ultimate veggie burger
    169–70
butternut squash: best-ever
  roast tomato soup 201

cabbage: mango and chilli
  salad 132
  quick pickled cabbage 147
  quick veg thoran 175–6
Cabbage Soup Diet 25
caffeine 93–4
calories 21, 25, 32, 49
cannellini beans: green
  minestrone 202
  tuna and white bean salad 126
  veggie two-bean chilli 166
caramelized onions 180
carbohydrates 36–7, 84, 95, 96
carrots: quick veg thoran 175–6
  ribbon vegetables 144

roast carrot and cumin
  dip 214
cashew and red chilli beef 136
casomorphins 94
cauliflower: hot roast
  vegetable curry 167–8
  veggie pilaf 180
cheese: flatbread pizzas 157
  hot green bean and feta
    salad 135
  ricotta, bananas and honey
    on rye toast 117
chewing food 24, 83
chicken 96
  chipotle chicken 147
  shredded cumin chicken 132
  smoked chicken and
    grapefruit cups 153
  steamed yoghurt chicken
    and cumin rice 160
  whole roast chicken 185–6
chickpeas: homemade
  hummus 210
chillies: chilli prawn cakes 144
  mango and chilli salad 132
  spicy hummus 212
  toasted cashew and red chilli
    beef 136
  veggie two-bean chilli 166
chipotle chicken 147
chocolate 58
Christmas 21, 23
coconut milk: quick coconut
  curry 139
  red lentil and coconut
    soup 196
cod: quick coconut curry 139
  roast cod with herby seed
    crust 165
  Spanish-style fish pie 171

coffee 97
comfort foods 35
conscious mind 18, 56, 64–5, 66, 72–3
convenience foods 36
coriander: salsas 148, 169–70
Cornell Food and Brand Lab 77
courgettes: flatbread pizzas 157
  veggie two-bean chilli 166
  green minestrone 202
  ribbon vegetables 144
  roasted vegetable and Puy lentil salad 128
crash diets 20
cravings 39, 84–5, 93
cream cheese: smoked fish pâté 209
cucumber: shredded salad 172
curry: curried parsnip mash 165
  hot roast vegetable curry 167–8
  quick coconut curry 139

dairy products 94, 95
dates: dairy-free date and apple porridge 109
  date squares 216
  fig, orange and pecan flapjacks 217
decision-making 17, 72–3
denial 42–3
destructive eaters 28, 33, 34, 37–8
diet diaries 47–8
diets 20, 24–7, 42
dinner plates, size 78–9
dinner tables 76–7
dips: homemade hummus 210

roast aubergine, lemon and garlic dip 213
roast carrot and cumin dip 214
roast tomato and rosemary hummus 212
spicy hummus 212
spicy peanut dipping sauce 151–2
dopamine 34
dried fruit 96
drinks: alcohol 84–5, 94, 95
  caffeine 87, 93–4, 97
  glass sizes 78–9
  herbal teas 97, 216
  smoothies 121–2

Easter 21
eaters, categories of 28–38
eating habits 48, 76–7, 82
eggs: huevos rancheros 108
  flat mushrooms with wilted spinach and poached eggs 110
  Scandi beetroot and smoked salmon mini frittata 154
  scrambled egg and tomato 111
  Vietnamese prawn omelette 137–8
emotional eaters 28, 30, 35
emotions 63
environmental factors 78–9
exercise 87
Eyton, Audrey 26

F-Plan diet 26
fasting 27
fat 39, 93
Fergusson, Dr Christy 13, 15, 73
fibre 26

fig, orange and pecan flapjacks 217
fish 96
  smoked fish pâté 209
  see also cod; salmon
5:2 diet 27
flapjacks: fig, orange and pecan 217
flatbread pizzas 157
Fletcher, Horace 24
food: cravings 39, 84, 93
  diaries 47–8
  labels 37, 93
  packaging 78–9
  proximity 80–1
  relationship with 23, 40
  'see food' trap 80–1
  shopping for 74, 75
food combining 25
frittata: Scandi beetroot and smoked salmon 154
fruit 97, 98
  berry and vanilla smoothie 122
  breakfast sundae 115
'fullness', recognizing 82–3

gastric bands 42
ghrelin 82
glucose 93
gluten 93
glycogen 84
granola 116
grapefruit: smoked chicken and grapefruit cups 153
green beans: green minestrone 202
  hot green bean and feta salad 135
  hot green salad 185–6

wholegrain green risotto 140
green minestrone 202
gut instincts 57–8

habits, changing 61–2, 94
habitual eaters 28, 31, 36
harissa prawns 192
Hay Diet 25
healthy-eating plan 100–3
herbal teas 97, 216
herbs 98
honey and wholegrain mustard
    roast salmon 182
hormones 82, 86
huevos rancheros 108
hummus 210
    roast tomato and rosemary
        hummus 212
    spicy hummus 212
hunger 74–5, 82
hypnosis 9, 11–12, 15, 17, 40–1,
    66–9

ignorant eaters 28, 32, 36–7
insulin 27, 37, 80

Japanese crunchy veg
    noodles 143
Johnson, Paul 39
junk food 39

kale: kale and roasted red veg
    salad 131
    kale crisps 206
    simple green smoothie 121
Kenny, Dr Paul 39
kidney beans: veggie two-
    bean chilli 166
Kinaesthetic Representational
    System 50, 52

king prawn and noodle stir
    fry 187–8

lactose intolerance 94
lamb tagine with potatoes
    and peas 189
lemon and dill bashed
    potatoes 182
lemon quinoa 192
lentils 96
    lentil and sweet potato stew
        179
    red lentil and coconut soup
        196
    roasted vegetable and
        Puy lentil salad 128
leptin 82–3
lime: apple and lime salsa 166
love, destructive eaters 37–8

mango and chilli salad 132
meal-replacement diet 26
mealtimes 76–7, 82
measuring yourself 45
meditation 87
melatonin 87
memories 40–1
metabolism 86
Mexican street food tacos 148
mind see brain; subconscious
    mind
mindful eating 83
mindful kitchen 96–8
minestrone, green 202
mint tea 216
mood boards 50, 59
Mosley, Dr Michael 27
muesli: blueberry and
    pistachio Bircher 118
mushrooms: flat mushrooms

with wilted spinach and
    poached eggs 110
ultimate veggie burger
    169–70

negative behaviour 63
negative thinking 47
Neuro Linguistic Programming
    (NLP) 50
neurotransmitters 34
Nidetch, Jean 26
noodles: Japanese crunchy
    veg noodles 143
    king prawn and noodle
        stir fry 187–8
nuts 96

oats: blueberry and pistachio
    Bircher 118
    dairy-free date and apple
        porridge 109
    fig, orange and pecan
        flapjacks 217
    no-sugar granola stash 116
oils 96
olive oil 96
omelette: Vietnamese prawn
    omelette 137–8
onions: caramelized onions 180
    Mexican street food tacos 148
oranges: fig, orange and pecan
    flapjacks 217
overeating: categories of
    eaters 28–39
    dinner plate size 78–9
    feeling of fullness 82–3
    triggers 28–33

packaging 78–9
pain 62

pak choi: toasted cashew
   and red chilli beef 136
   Vietnamese prawn omelette
   137–8
pancakes, smoked salmon and
   spinach 112
Parma ham, pea and
   watercress soup with 198
parsnips: curried parsnip
   mash 165
pasta: my favourite ragu with
   spelt pasta 162
pâté, smoked fish 209
Pavlov's dogs 80
peanut dipping sauce 151–2
peas: green minestrone 202
   hot green salad 185–6
   lemon quinoa 192
   pea and watercress soup 198
   wasabi salmon and peas 177
   wholegrain green risotto 140
pecan nuts: fig, orange and
   pecan flapjacks 217
Peer, Marisa 9–12, 15, 28, 61
peppers: flatbread pizzas 157
   huevos rancheros 108
   kale and roasted red veg
   salad 131
   roasted vegetable and
   Puy lentil salad 128
   tuna and white bean salad 126
   veggie two-bean chilli 166
Peters, Lulu Hunt 25
photos, before-and-after 45
pilaf, veggie 180
pistachio nuts: blueberry and
   pistachio Bircher 118
pizzas, flatbread 157
planning meals 74–5
plates, size 78–9

pleasure 62
porridge, dairy-free date
   and apple 109
portion control 78–9
positive thinking 47
potatoes: lamb tagine with
   potatoes and peas 189
   lemon and dill bashed
   potatoes 182
   Spanish-style fish pie 171
prawns: chilli prawn cakes 144
   king prawn and noodle stir
   fry 187–8
   spicy harissa prawns 192
   Vietnamese prawn omelette
   137–8
   Vietnamese summer rolls
   151–2
pre-ordering meals 74–5
Preferred Representational
   Systems 50–2
processed foods 95
pulses 96
pumpkin seeds: date
   squares 216
   no-sugar granola stash 116

quinoa, lemon 192

radishes: Japanese crunchy
   veg noodles 143
ragu, my favourite 162
raisins: no-sugar granola
   stash 116
ready meals 36
red cabbage: quick pickled
   cabbage 147
regression, timeline 40–1
Representational Systems
   50–2

restaurants 75
ribbon vegetables 144
rice: quick coconut curry 139
   steamed yoghurt chicken
   and cumin rice 160
   veggie pilaf 180
   wholegrain green risotto 140
ricotta, bananas and honey on
   rye toast 117
risotto, wholegrain green 140
rye toast see toast

salads: hot green bean
   and feta salad 135
   hot green salad 185–6
   kale and roasted red veg
   salad 131
   mango and chilli salad 132
   roasted vegetable and
   Puy lentil salad 128
   shredded salad 172
   spicy tomato salad 160
   tuna and white bean
   salad 126
salmon: honey and wholegrain
   mustard roast salmon 182
   speedy Thai-style salmon
   190
   tandoori fish 175–6
   wasabi salmon and peas 177
salsa 169–70
   apple and lime salsa 166
   quick coriander salsa 148
salt 84
Scandi beetroot and smoked
   salmon mini frittata 154
second helpings 82–3
Secret Eaters 12–13, 42, 73,
   76, 83, 86
'see food' trap 80–1

seeds 96
  toasted seeds 203
Selfridges 42–3
senses 72
shopping 74–5
sleep 86–7
Slim Fast Diet 26
slimming clubs 26, 43
smoked chicken and
  grapefruit cups 153
smoked fish pâté 209
smoked salmon: Scandi
  beetroot and smoked
  salmon mini frittata 154
  smoked salmon and spinach
  spelt pancakes 112
smoking 58
smoothies: berry and vanilla
  smoothie 122
  simple green smoothie 121
snacks 76–7
sodium 84
soups: best-ever roast tomato
  soup 201
  green minestrone 202
  pea and watercress soup 198
  red lentil and coconut soup
  196
  sweet potato soup 203
soya milk: dairy-free date and
  apple porridge 109
Spanish-style fish pie 171
spelt pancakes, smoked salmon
  and spinach 112
spelt pasta, my favourite ragu
  with 162
spinach: flat mushrooms with
  wilted spinach and
  poached eggs 110
  smoked salmon and spinach

spelt pancakes 112
simple green smoothie 121
  wholegrain green risotto 140
Stanford Hypnotic
  Susceptibility Scales 67
stew, lentil and sweet potato
  179
stimulants 95
stir fries: green veg stir fry 190
  king prawn and noodle stir
  fry 187–8
subconscious mind 17, 18,
  56–69
  changing habits 61–2
  destructive eaters 37
  and emotions 63
  hypnosis 66–9
  negative thinking 47
  pain and pleasure 62
  visualization 59
  and willpower 64–5
sugar 39, 93, 95, 97
sugar snap peas: Japanese
  crunchy veg noodles 143
summer rolls, Vietnamese 151–2
sundae, breakfast 115
sunflower seeds: no-sugar
  granola stash 116
sunlight 87
Supersize v Superskinny 8–11,
  43
sweet potatoes: lentil and
  sweet potato stew 179
  sweet potato soup 203
  ultimate veggie burger
  169–70
  wasabi salmon and peas with
  roasted sweet potato 177
sweeteners 95, 97
tacos, Mexican street food 148

tagine, lamb 189
tandoori fish 175–6
teas 98
  mint tea 216
temptation 80–1
Thai-style salmon 190
thoran, quick veg 175–6
timeline regression 40–1
tinned food 96
tiredness 86–7
toast: avocado and bacon on
  rye toast 106
  ricotta, bananas and honey
  on rye toast 117
  scrambled egg and tomato
  on rye toast 111
tofu: Japanese crunchy veg
  noodles 143
tomatoes: best-ever roast
  tomato soup 201
  huevos rancheros 108
  kale and roasted red veg
  salad 131
  roast tomato and rosemary
  hummus 212
  salsas 148, 169–70
  scrambled egg and tomato
  111
  Spanish-style fish pie 171
  spicy tomato salad 160
  tuna and white bean salad 126
  my favourite ragu with spelt
  pasta 162
  veggie two-bean chilli 166
tortillas: flatbread pizzas 157
trances, hypnosis 66
triggers, overeating 28–33
tuna and white bean salad 126
TVs 76–7, 87
20-minute rule 82–3

simple green smoothie 121
my favourite ragu with spelt
	pasta 162
ultimate veggie burger 169–70

vegetables 97, 98
	ribbon vegetables 144
	veggie pilaf 180
	veggie two-bean chilli 166
	see also peppers, tomatoes
		etc
Vietnamese prawn omelette
	137–8
Vietnamese summer rolls 151–2
Visual Representational System
	50, 51
visualization exercises 59
vitamin D 87

wasabi salmon and peas 177
watercress: pea and watercress
	soup 198
weighing yourself 43–4
Weight Watchers 26
wheat 93
wholegrain green risotto 140
willpower 64–5, 80

'yo-yo' weight loss 20
yoghurt: breakfast sundae 115
	roast aubergine, lemon and
		garlic dip 213
	steamed yoghurt chicken
		and cumin rice 160

Zone Diet 27

REFERENCES

The experiments in Step Two came from the following sources:

Calvin A. D., R. E. Carter , T. Adachi , P. G. Macedo , F. N. Albuquerque , C. van der Walt, J. Bukartyk, D. E. Davison , J. A. Levine , V. K. Somers: 'Effects of experimental sleep restriction on caloric intake and activity energy expenditure'. Chest. 2013 Jul;144(1):79–86. doi: 10.1378/chest.12-2829.

Hanks, Andrew S., David R. Just and Brian Wansink: 'Preordering school lunch encourages better food choices by children'. Journal of the American Medical Association: Pediatrics 167.7 (2013): 673–674.

Society for the Study of Ingestive Behavior: 'Ghrelin increases willingness to pay for food'. ScienceDaily, 15 July 2011.

Tal, Aner, Scott Zuckerman and Brian Wansink: 'Watch what you eat: TV content influences consumption'. Journal of the American Medical Association: Internal Medicine, 2014 doi:10.1001/jamainternmed.2014.4098.

Wansink, Brian: 'Can package size accelerate usage volume?'. Journal of Marketing, July 1996, 60:3, 1–14.

Wansink, Brian: Mindless Eating: Why We Eat More Than We Think. New York, NY: Bantam Dell, 2006.

Wansink Brian, J. E. Painter, J.E. Lee YK: 'The office candy dish: proximity's influence on estimated and actual consumption'. Int J Obes (London). 2006 May, 30(5):871–5.

Yeomans, M. R.: 'Short term effects of alcohol on appetite in humans: effects of context and restrained eating'. Appetite, 2010, 55(3), 565–573

★ ★ ★

A BIG THANK YOU

★ ★ ★

Bringing a book to life from pitch to page requires a team with creative genius, focus and passion in their blood. I'm lucky to have worked with the best. It's a little thing, but thank you says so very much...

The Wordsmiths
Thank you to Deputy Publishing Director Sarah Emsley at Headline for fronting such an enthusiastic team, and being the essence of calm and charm throughout. To our magnificent editor, Emma Tait – you take Auditory Digital to a whole new level and I love you for it. Thank you. Georgina Moore, your press strategy (and phone voice) has left me a little giddy – I don't know whether to thank you or stalk you. And of course, I wouldn't have met any of you without Charlotte Robertson at United Agents – thanks Charlotte, you were a gift.

The Artists
This is a beautiful book – my heartfelt thanks to the team at Smith & Gilmour for making it so. Matt Russell, your photography is as gorgeous as your manner, thank you. And to my dear pal and make-up artist Clare Turner, I'd be a bit lost (and a whole lot uglier) without you. You went above and beyond, you star.

The Foodies
Huge thanks to Louisa Carter, Charlotte Simpkins and Emma Marsden for creating and styling such astonishingly lovely recipes. I'm sorry I ate everything on the shoot...

The Experts
I owe a huge debt of gratitude to hypnotherapist Marisa Peer and psychologist Dr Christy Fergusson whose collaboration was essential in the creation of this book. Every time I work with you, it's a real pleasure – thank you to both of you.

And finally...
None of this would have happened had I not been lucky enough to have worked with Colette Foster and her team at Remarkable Television, or indeed the features commissioning team at Channel 4. Thank you, too, to Cognitive Hypnotherapist Trevor Silvester who is patiently training me in hypnotherapy as we speak.

Last but not least, my love and thanks to Snoop... always.